AT THE LIMITS OF CARE

Gendered Work and Stories That Matter

For author Janna Klostermann, reaching her limits and resigning from care work felt like a crisis of self. In the aftermath of this upheaval, this is the book she needed to write. *At the Limits of Care* will change how you think about care work and about the women who provide it.

Now an assistant professor in sociology and a radical care scholar, Klostermann interrogates women's counter stories of reaching their limits, crossing ethical lines, and stepping back from paid or unpaid care work roles. She weaves feminist sociological analyses with memoir to challenge dominant narratives around women and care, transforming the ways we think about ourselves and our relationships.

The book makes a major contribution in how and what constitutes care research. Drawing on in-depth life history interviews with women ages twenty-seven to seventy-eight in Ontario, Canada, Klostermann enacts a "counter politics of care" approach that centres untold and lesser-told stories of care work. She pushes readers to rethink gendered power dynamics, question prevailing tropes of care, and imagine more equitable, emancipatory futures.

JANNA KLOSTERMANN is an assistant professor in the Department of Sociology at the University of Calgary.

At the Limits of Care

Gendered Work and Stories That Matter

JANNA KLOSTERMANN

UNIVERSITY OF TORONTO PRESS
Toronto Buffalo London

© University of Toronto Press 2025
Toronto Buffalo London
utppublishing.com
Printed in the USA

ISBN 978-1-4875-6394-3 (cloth)   ISBN 978-1-4875-6397-4 (EPUB)
ISBN 978-1-4875-6395-0 (paper)   ISBN 978-1-4875-6396-7 (PDF)

Library and Archives Canada Cataloguing in Publication

Title: At the limits of care : gendered work and stories that matter /
    Janna Klostermann.
Names: Klostermann, Janna, author.
Description: Includes bibliographical references and index.
Identifiers: Canadiana (print) 20250197189 | Canadiana (ebook)
    20250197197 | ISBN 9781487563943 (cloth) | ISBN 9781487563950
    (paper) | ISBN 9781487563974 (EPUB) | ISBN 9781487563967 (PDF)
Subjects: LCSH: Women caregivers – Ontario. | LCSH: Feminism.
Classification: LCC HQ1459.O57 K56 2025 | DDC 305.409713 – dc23

Cover design: Val Cooke
Cover images: iStock.com/CSA-Printstock; iStock.com/tolgart

We wish to acknowledge the land on which the University of Toronto
Press operates. This land is the traditional territory of the Wendat, the
Anishnaabeg, the Haudenosaunee, the Métis, and the Mississaugas of the
Credit First Nation.

This book has been published with the help of a grant from the Federation
for the Humanities and Social Sciences, through the Awards to Scholarly
Publications Program, using funds provided by the Social Sciences and
Humanities Research Council of Canada.

University of Toronto Press acknowledges the financial support of the
Government of Canada, the Canada Council for the Arts, and the Ontario
Arts Council, an agency of the Government of Ontario, for its publishing
activities.

Canada Council   Conseil des Arts
for the Arts   du Canada

ONTARIO ARTS COUNCIL
CONSEIL DES ARTS DE L'ONTARIO
an Ontario government agency
un organisme du gouvernement de l'Ontario

Funded by the   Financé par le
Government   gouvernement
of Canada   du Canada

Canadä

To Claire, Kathy, Gail, and Irene

Contents

Acknowledgments

This book has undergone multiple revisions, as I've come to tell fuller stories about my experiences and struggles as a care worker. Somewhere along the way, it sunk in that my interest in the "limits of care" wasn't just about loss or how much was taken from me, but about the magnitude of my love. Grief is like that, I think. Writing "at the limits" – that is, writing this book and playing my edge – has helped me to get somewhere, and I am incredibly grateful for the many ways I've been supported and sustained along the way.

This research was generously supported by a SSHRC Joseph-Armand Bombardier Canada Graduate Scholarship, as well as by two Ontario Graduate Scholarships. It has benefited from institutional support and funding at Carleton University where I completed my PhD in Sociology, Brock University where I held a SSHRC postdoctoral fellowship in Sociology, and the University of Calgary where I am currently an assistant professor in Sociology. I'm grateful to have served as a visiting scholar in Maastricht University's Arts, Media and Culture Programme, and as a resident fellow in the Calgary Institute for the Humanities.

First and foremost, thank you to my PhD supervisor, Susan Braedley. I am incredibly grateful for you encouraging me to say what is mine to say and pointing to what's possible in community. I am also grateful to my doctoral committee members Janet Siltanen and Megan Rivers-Moore, and to examiners Rebecca Schein and Laura Funk. I have learned so much collaborating with other care labour and aging studies scholars on powerhouse research teams led by Drs. Pat Armstrong, Sally Chivers, Tamara Daly, Andrea Doucet, and Laura Funk. At the University of Calgary, I have been grateful to work with wonderful colleagues and students. Thank you all! To Saro Bunting, I am still singing your praises for your editorial support, and for you asking me, "shouldn't you at least tell the reader about your formative religious upbringing or initial draw into care work?"

Thanks also to my colleagues and writing buddies in Ottawa and beyond for investing in me and in this project. I'm particularly grateful to my "co-worker" Taylor Winfield, to members of the "ass in chair" writing group – Susanne Fletcher, Sharon Hamilton, and Catherine Racine – and to members of the "farties" writing group – Katherine Occhiuto, Anna Przednowek, and Christine Streeter. Thank you to my colleagues who showed up to talk shop, read drafts, or set a timer to write in shared silence together: Britt Amell, Nina Doré, Chloë Grace Fogarty-Bourget, Zoey Jones, Samantha McAleese, Lauren Montgomery, Sarah Rodimon, Valerie Stam, Tara McWhinney, and Amanda Van Beinum. Thanks also to my dear friends Sharon Caldwell, Emily Grant, Stef Hogan, Jillian Kennedy, and Kim Radford.

Many thanks to the women who contributed to this research, and to those I worked with and supported at L'Arche and the group home. My work as a care worker, and as a care scholar, has kept me on the edge of my seat, and I'm grateful for how much I've been learning in conversation and community. Thank you to all who've accompanied me.

I also wish to thank the University of Toronto Press for their interest in this book, and generous support along the way. A huge thank you to acquisitions editor Jodi Lewchuck – a feminist memoirist in her own right – for "getting" the project and seeing the power of it. Thanks also to Janice Evans for guiding the book through the production process, to Melissa MacAulay for copy-editing, to Siusan Moffat for generating the index, and to Val Cooke for the cover design. I am also grateful to Kelly Laycock for her careful review of the manuscript, and to three anonymous reviewers for their deep engagement and intellectual generosity.

A heartfelt thanks to my family who taught me how to set up a story, land a joke, and push for something more. I wouldn't be where I am without you, Mom and Dad. Much love to Nanny and Ga, and to Claire, Brandon, Trevor, Ty, and Rossi. I'm grateful for all the family theatrics. To my partner, Philip, thank you! I recently came across a message you sent me while we both lived and worked at L'Arche that said, "If you can write about it, you'll start feeling better I think." I don't think you expected I'd be writing for another ten years, but there was something to your advice, and I'm grateful you've been up for one adventure after another.

Honestly, thanks.

AT THE LIMITS OF CARE

Care Junkie Diaries: The Memoir

Starting at the Limits

At the limits of care, I met the criteria on every burn-out, compassion fatigue, or nervous breakdown test I could find online. I had every sign and symptom of extreme emotional distress. Persistently sad and hopeless. Guilty, worthless, ashamed. Irritable and moody. Self-destructive, sensitive to criticism, overwhelmed by life. I was wound right up – dragging my body from task to task and room to room, but not quite thinking straight. It was remarkable how limited my resources were, how hopeless I felt, but I'm not sure if it was just burn-out or depletion, or if any of those clinical-sounding terms cut it. It seemed like a descent. A darkness that I couldn't see out of. Something even more dismantling than can be put into words.

It's hard to tell when my lowest point was, or when things started to go sideways.

It could have been when I took a full week off from care work, until I could stop crying long enough to return. That was around the time that I remember crying to a friend in a sloppy, out-of-control way in a Starbucks in the suburbs. It was enough for the guy beside us to get up and head to the other side of the coffee shop, which disappointed me a great deal at the time, as I thought maybe I had his ear, that he might have been impressed by how I was putting it.

I started off so well-meaning. I really did. I was hungry for something to latch on to, to live a life of purpose.

When I first landed a job as a support worker at a residential group home, it felt like a privilege to be there. At the job interview, I remember meeting two adults with developmental disabilities who spoke American Sign Language. I introduced myself by signing my own name. J-A-N-N-A was all I knew. Not knowing any more than that felt symbolic, a sign that I was being called beyond myself. Much like how Peace Corps volunteers narrate themselves as infantile, dependent, ignorant, or helpless upon arrival (Schein 2008), I put the emphasis on my own incompetence and ignorance, on how much I wanted to decentre myself to listen and learn from others.

From the start, I hit it off with my co-workers and with the disabled residents we supported at the group home. The job involved making meals, doing laundry, cleaning the house, and supporting with personal, social, and emotional care. I enjoyed painting nails, organizing Tupperware drawers, and going for jogs with the wheelchair users I supported. One resident had one of those adaptive wheelchair bikes; I used to *sprint* alongside him and tease him that he shouldn't be driving drunk. He didn't drink, but raised me an imaginary one, cupping his hand in the air, as he weaved along the bike path, laughing. As the self-proclaimed "rec girl," I enjoyed loading others into the wheelchair van to hit up parks, bookstores, coffee shops, and dive bars. Co-workers and I raced to the punchline, pretending to suffer groin injuries or to doze off mid-conversation only to have others wake us up. I once walked into work dressed as a bowl of grapes with a dozen purple balloons tied to me. Some commented that I brought out a funnier, light-hearted side of the people we supported. I felt the work was doing the same for me.

Prior to the group home job, I had studied at Roberts Wesleyan College, a small-town liberal arts Christian college in upstate New York, for undergrad. After graduation, I spent an entire year volunteering full-time as part of an urban service corps program in Los Angeles. During that service year, I worked at a homeless service centre in Venice Beach and lived in a church rectory in Inglewood with five other young adults. I felt called to a life of service. But when I first moved home from LA to Peterborough, Ontario, in the summer of 2008, at age twenty-three, I handed out two dozen résumés, only to hear crickets. No one wanted me. In a recession and in a city with one of the highest unemployment rates in Canada, Country Style Donuts was the only job I could find.

When I finally got that job at the group home, almost a year later at age twenty-four, I was over the moon. I considered it my first real adult job; it meant something, and I got paid. After having spent my teens and early twenties immersed in Christian or unitarian-ish social justice teachings and communities, working at the group home seemed like the ideal way to live out my faith. At the time, I was pursuing a master's in pastoral studies online at Loyola University Chicago, where I took courses that had through lines about living out visions of emancipatory political transformation, unsettling dominant norms, going where our gladness meets the world's need. I was awed by teachings that seemed to point to what was possible in community. I too wanted to connect beyond difference, to live in right relation with myself and others.

At the group home, I remember feeling honoured the first time I applied one woman's evening foot cream. It wasn't that I thought of myself as a Mary Magdalene type, washing Jesus's feet. I wasn't devout in that way. But I teared up a little, thinking there were lessons in the work for me, ways that I was being invited to acknowledge truths about the human condition or our shared need for care. I also felt honoured when I accompanied a resident while he was in the ICU with a breathing tube and with IVs and tape all over him. I held his hand and put ChapStick on his dry lips. It felt like a privilege to be with him and so fully in the moment. It was as if someone had drawn a circle in the sand around me. *No where else to be, nowhere else to go.*

As a support worker, I liked working the 3:00 p.m. to 9:00 p.m. shift, as it meant that I could hit up bars with co-workers and friends afterwards. I went out a few nights a week and saw it as a way to "keep an even keel" or put myself first after working long, full shifts serving others. I enjoyed going out with co-workers and introducing the disabled people I supported to friends outside work. I remember meeting up with a co-worker after our shifts to talk about our life goals and who we were becoming. Care work was part of that process of self-discovery too. I can also remember hanging out in a park with a few residents, as a friend strummed her ukulele, and we all sipped iced tea. The lines between work and non-work were blurry, and I liked that.

I also liked that the job came with a built-in sense of community. I was proud to be part of the downtown Peterborough social justice scene, and proud to work alongside so many artists, activists, and former women's studies majors. Co-workers and I talked a lot about disability politics, power-sharing, turning towards others. We took turns sharing recipes for soups with a Moroccan twist or homemade pizzas where you mix goat cheese in with the pizza sauce. Even mundane aspects of the work felt meaningful. I couldn't believe what a game-changer that goat cheese was, how I was getting paid to try things like that.

It was hard to see, at first, what an under-resourced organization I was at. It was precarious part-time work. I was glad to make around eighteen bucks an hour at a time when rent was affordable in Peterborough. And I didn't mind being on call or occasionally working split shifts, two hours in the morning and five hours in the evening. But I found it hard to walk on eggshells. In my first year of working at the group home, "Tonya,"[1] the manager of our home, fired four or five of my co-workers. It seemed the more someone invested, the higher their chances were of being let go. The writing was on the wall for me. This was all too clear when Tonya announced, at a staff meeting, that she was *banning* any form of comedy, humour, or joking around in the workplace or in staff meetings in particular. She looked over at me as she made the announcement. "I think she's threatened by your humour," a co-worker commented after. "She sees how disruptive it can be, how you use it to bring people together."

I had to wonder if I'd pushed it too far with the odd joke about our untenable working conditions. When a co-worker popped a blood vessel in his eye, I teased in a team meeting that we should all pop a vessel in the name of the care – throw out our backs in the name of community. I also once jokingly addressed our executive director with "Hey, big boy!" He laughed, and it seemed kind of folksy and endearing at the time, but perhaps it had been too much?

I didn't regret any of that though. I mostly just pitied Tonya for trying to claim power where there was none to be had. Every rule she came up with seemed like a power grab or a way to take the fun out of the work. There was the "no comedy" rule, the "no changing shifts without going through her so *she* could decide who *she* wanted to give those hours to" rule, and the "no making recipes that weren't on her menu" rule. When I saw Tuna Casserole Tuesdays on the calendar, I couldn't help but feel for the residents. The way Tonya "managed" us, and the ways that we were to "manage" the people we supported, left something to be desired. I hated that our job involved reading out a rule book to a disabled guy in his forties – reminding him that we were staff, *not* his friends. I didn't agree with

---

1 Note: pseudonyms are used throughout the book, with the exception of some friends, colleagues, or mentors whom I mention by name. When it comes to ethical issues around representation, I cheered to read an "Author's Note" by Amanda Montei (2023) that captured my own approach to memoir writing quite beautifully. She writes: "Women receive an undue burden when it comes to remembering. This is especially true when they choose to tell stories about violation and patriarchal control. This is a work of nonfiction. Some names and identifying details have been changed to protect the identities of characters ... Conversations have been reconstructed from memory and some events have been compressed for readability. Like all memoir, the personal recollections contained herein have also been reshaped by time, memory, and the craft of writing. They are no less true" (xii). From her point about how hard it is to tell stories about violation and patriarchal control to her description of the writing, editing, and reconstructing process, she captures my own approach well. I will reflect in future chapters on my process and on how our stories change over time. In the meantime, I join her in saying that reconstructed stories are no less true.

the approach and didn't think there was anything wrong with befriending others or finding more mutual ways of providing support.

The more I read about L'Arche, a community where people with and without disabilities live together as equals, the more I thought it could be an ideal next step for me.

In his book *Finding Peace*, Jean Vanier (2003), the founder of L'Arche, wrote about the value of building community across difference and about how he had committed his life to honouring people with intellectual and developmental disabilities, living in community with them. When I first encountered Vanier's work, I didn't realize he was a serial sex offender who had abused live-in caregivers, as that part wasn't public knowledge yet.[2] I truly thought he was on to something, with over 150 L'Arche communities around the world. As I read his book, I wrote "Love it" in the margins of multiple pages. I felt called to work for peace and to make peace with the parts of myself I'd rejected.

I loved the spiritual invitation to share life on the arc, build relationships across difference, and reveal the unique value and vocation of each individual. I thought the organization's focus on helping people *with and without disabilities* bring forth their unique gifts would serve me well. The fact that the job provided room and board attracted to me too, as part of me didn't want to grow up too quickly. The year before, when a friend had suggested that we should get an apartment together, even that was too much. *And furnish it? Pay hydro?* I recoiled. I didn't want life to come at me too hard.

I was thrilled to hand in my resignation letter at the group home, and thrilled to submit my application to live and serve at L'Arche. *So long, Tonya!*

Ship of Fools?

I felt called to community life when I first interviewed for the position of live-in assistant at L'Arche – a position that involved working split shifts, mornings and evenings, sixty-odd hours a week in exchange for

---

2 In March of 2020, Jean Vanier was credibly accused of emotionally and sexually abusing six women, including live-in care workers, under the guise of "spiritual accompaniment." In an internal inquiry by L'Arche, Vanier was described as initiating manipulative and coercive sex with multiple women. After hearing the news about the alleged abuses, I published an op-ed in the *Toronto Star* to elaborate on how the power structure at L'Arche makes young workers vulnerable to exploitation (Klostermann 2020). That part of my story will become clearer as we go. I will also revisit the news of the scandal in the interlude between chapters 5 and 6.

room, board, and a stipend. I felt special in the L'Arche job interview – like I mattered. They asked about my favourite books and movies, about who I was and what I desired. They complimented my comic sensibilities *and* my spiritual commitments. They hinted that they could see me like no one else could see me, and that L'Arche would be an ideal space to make myself vulnerable and express my unique gifts. They prodded at my desire to be good, pointing me in the direction of moral worth.

I have never had an employer take such an interest in me – in the real me. The me I prefer to talk about. I was thrilled to mention that I had taken the stage at every talent show or open mic night in high school and university, that I'd even performed at a few open mic comedy nights in LA. I loved how much they saw in me, and imagined I'd be as wildly alive and in my spiritual glory at L'Arche, as I had been during my undergrad in Rochester and during that year of service in LA. To me, L'Arche seemed like the ideal way to commit to an ethical life. I liked the promise that if we surrender to community life, there'd be a joy or an energy that's freed up.

After the interview, I walked from the main office to one of the L'Arche homes where disabled adults, known as "core members," live alongside caregivers known as "live-in assistants." I wanted to make a good impression, to show that I'd be a caring addition to community life. I offered to set the table for dinner but was told it was someone else's job. During dinner, I went to help serve dessert but was told that was someone else's job too. At the end of the meal, I tried to clear the table and was again told that it was someone else's job. They eventually let me load the dishwasher, but only after one of them explained that the beauty of community life was that each person had a unique way to contribute. It wasn't about being the most caring or the quickest to help but about slowing down to share space with others. Everyone had a part to play.

In *The Disabled God*, Nancy Eiesland (1994) writes, "Often our bone-weariness with living a difficult life made more difficult by stigmatizing social systems necessitates that we rebel" (95). It was a sentence I underlined around the time of moving into L'Arche. I didn't want a baby or a bungalow or a professional life, and thought of myself as taking a rebellious counter path by pursuing care as a vocation. Jeanette Winterson (1996) writes, "The artist cannot occupy middle ground, and the warm nooks of humanity are not for her, she lives on the mountainside, in the desert, on the sea. The condition of the artist is a condition of Remove" (168). When I first read the quote, I thought she described my situation perfectly. I was an artist, for sure;

I also thought my height had something to do with that "condition of Remove" she references.

As a six-foot-three woman, I grew up playing my gender role in an unconventional way in small-town Ontario. I wasn't going to marry a Peterborough Petes hockey player, so I worked on my funny bone instead. Louise Bernikow (1980) writes that "whether a female is 'pretty' or not is crucial to the story" (6). At my height, I wasn't expecting to be taken care of by a man or to fold into a normative professional path. Instead, from a young age, I carved out a counter path, seeking out the margins. L'Arche seemed liked another way to do that. As my friends from high school and college were rushing to get married, get good jobs, and have kids, being part of an international movement centred on caring and communal living seemed like a promising alternative. It seemed like a way to continue building a life around difference. My desire for class mobility was part of the pull too. As the daughter of an autoworker and the first in my family to go to college, I cheered at the number of writers and thinkers with master's degrees who lived and worked at L'Arche. It felt like a classed, intellectual project of sorts. A way to go after a big life.

On my first morning as a live-in assistant, I woke up at 6:30 a.m. to start my 6:45 shift. I quickly brushed my teeth and hair and changed my clothes. When I stepped onto the main floor of the house, I delighted to hear Lori, one of the residents with a disability, *sprinting* towards me. I heard her run through the kitchen, down the hall, and around and into the living room. I braced myself for a greeting of a lifetime, only for her to look up, see it was me, and disappointedly say, "Oh, just you." There was an edge to how she said it. I had to laugh that she couldn't even be bothered to say hello, that there was nothing revelatory or remotely friendly about it. *Wasn't that what Vanier had promised?* Part of me liked being put in my place though. I took it as a reminder that the relationships worth building are the hard-won ones, that we need to work for things. I was also certain Lori and I would be hitting it off in no time, that she'd see my fun-loving, goofy side, see how much I was investing.

In the first L'Arche home that I lived in, there were eight people, including four core members and four live-in assistants from around the world. I worked with assistants from Canada, Brazil, Bulgaria, Germany, the Philippines, Korea, and Ukraine, including several who had moved to Canada in hopes of applying for permanent residency status. The first home that I lived in was one of several L'Arche homes in that particular community, and the community I lived in was one of over

150 L'Arche communities worldwide, and not the one that the founder, Vanier, lived in.[3]

"Slowing down to make the joke, rather than rushing through the motions" is how I described my life as a live-in assistant. I embraced the slow pace of routines and prided myself in doing ordinary work with reverence. I thought of myself as "being," not "doing" or "striving." Similar to the group home, my main duties were to provide support with personal care, medications, meals, and general friendship and fun. I made roasted red pepper soup, beer bread, and espresso cake. I liked French-braiding hair and helping others pick out stylish outfits. I operated the Hoyer lift to transfer a woman I supported from her wheelchair into the bathtub; I also sat with her while she bathed in case she had a seizure. I enjoyed initiating outings or offering to drive when others made plans. I even found a nice groove with Lori. She pronounced my name "Shanna," and greeted me and others warmly when we entered the room. "Shanna, you lucky, girl," she said. "That Shanna, she lucky."

From the start, life at L'Arche felt loaded with meaning, like everything had a hidden message I could decipher. I wrote it down when Krista, a disabled woman I lived with, said, "God is the only hope we have," to which Lori responded, "I'm right here, you yo-yo." I thought there was wisdom in that. I myself had pursued a life of service because I wanted to experience the presence of God in community. I had long given up on the idea of an all-powerful God that was outside of us or "up there," so I liked the way Lori put it. I also wrote it down when, after being wished a happy forty-first birthday, Krista said, "Thanks; I don't look it." I made a note in my journal about how she was resisting societal expectations around what it means to be a certain age, how I myself was travelling by story, learning in dialogue.

I was all in on all fronts, actively making something of it.

At L'Arche, I didn't feel like I was on a ship of fools searching for that which cannot be found. The beer in the fridge felt like the perfect example; it didn't seem like an otherworldly, overly polished, prefigurative, idyllic community, but rather one in which there might be space for something "real," space to connect across difference with people from around the world who were committing to the making of a better world. I enjoyed what I called "the ebb and flow of daily living" and the conversations along the way. My house leader was fun to be

---

3 I lived in two different L'Arche communities over the course of two and a half years. For the purposes of this memoir, I have combined the two homes, changed all names, and changed some identifying details.

in the room with, good at creating space for intimacy and intellectuality among women. She encouraged us as we swapped philosophical insights in team meetings and packed our bags for the odd road trip. She was good at noticing others' needs and what we were saying with our lives. At L'Arche, living with so many young adults was part of the fun too. I enjoyed the retreats and "meeting hall" parties with other live-in assistants. I particularly enjoyed hanging out with Philip, a live-in assistant from Germany, whom I started dating shortly after I moved in and got married to shortly after I resigned.

Something about being at L'Arche felt like a way to go after a good life story, to do something unique and interesting with my life. I liked being taken care of too. I liked that there were sleeves of bagels in the pantry, that everything from our meals to our housing and vehicle maintenance was taken care of. We used the gas card to fill up the tank, and we were even allowed to buy wine for special occasions. At the time, I occasionally thought about what my life would be like if I chased my wildest dreams and pursued a master of fine arts in creative writing, but I didn't get much further than reading the bios of faculty members online, as I couldn't get over what a lonely path that would be. I pictured myself holed up in a dingy Montreal studio apartment with an air mattress, chain-smoking. I didn't smoke but imagined I'd resort to it if I was cut off from the kind of creative inspiration I was having in community.

It was a weird feeling, and hard to describe, but I can remember feeling contained or held in place when I first started as a live-in worker. To get to my bedroom I had to go through the laundry room and past a utility sink, stand-alone shower, and second fridge. The room had low ceilings, bare walls, a twin bed, and a view of the wheelchair van in the driveway. As a six-foot-three woman, folding into such a tiny room felt symbolic. As a writer, a bite-sized desk that I couldn't write at was the cherry on top. I felt like I was stripping everything away from my life – all that didn't matter – to build a life of purpose. I was switching from a showboat-y "Janna show" to humble work in community. There was a clear map for how to live a moral life, a routine to hold me in place. I could catch on.

Moral Cards

There was pleasure in the learning curve. Co-workers and I talked about how to cultivate relationships that respected difference, making space for the people we supported. I can remember helping to put a stop to condescending pet names or to some co-workers ordering lunch for core members without involving them. I intervened when an eighteen-year-old guy tried to cheer up an older woman we supported, saying, "*Aww,* honey, you know everyone loves you, right?" He *purred* as he spoke, and I thought it sounded infantilizing coming from him. I enjoyed noticing things that could be done differently and considering whether or how to respond. Fellow live-in assistants also coached me in "entering the world" of the people we supported, discerning their expressions and offers. One co-worker suggested that each time I came on shift, I should kneel or crouch on the floor to greet a core member who used a wheelchair but preferred to crawl around at home – to give her a warm, personalized welcome, rather than saying hello while standing above her. "Enter *her* world," my co-worker said.

Good, bad. Right, wrong. I defined myself through those boundaries.

I learned not to use the word "work" to describe living with and supporting people, and not to write "Holly was good today" in the communications book. Saying "Holly had a good day" was one thing, but to evaluate her on some scale of being "well-behaved" was quite another. We also resisted the urge to use pathologizing language or to talk about the complex psychiatric diagnoses or rather profound needs of some of the people we supported. We were taught to focus on the "friendships" we were building, rather than the skills needed to support core members who were showing signs of dementia or who had been diagnosed with autism, schizophrenia, Down syndrome, or other conditions.

With fine-grained status distinctions at play, we had "full days," instead of busy or burdensome ones. We also took "time away" instead of "time off." The word "off," we were told, made it sound like labour, as though we thought the disabled people we lived with were a lot of work. Two women I supported were fully incontinent and non-verbal, which meant that we helped to do "check-ins" to change their diapers every couple of hours, several times a day. We squeezed into bathroom stalls in coffee shops and community centres. On one occasion, I even took off my own tights (that I had under a short dress) so that the woman I was with could have something dry to wear. I got better at interpreting hand motions and facial expressions and at remembering to restock the backpack with supplies and a change of pants.

When women in Starbucks charged over to compliment me or other live-in assistants for being "angels" or for not knowing how we did it, we were quick to say that we were the lucky ones for getting to hang out with the people we supported, that they were the "angels" for putting up with us. We prided ourselves in saying the moral thing, distinguishing our moral approaches from those of others.

At team meetings, we occasionally talked about how the parents of the people we supported hadn't been able to hack it. One put her daughter in a group home from a young age. Another faked a cancer scare to get his daughter bumped to the top of the L'Arche wait-list. There was also the couple who reportedly used to lock their daughter in the attic, dropping her off to her day program dishevelled and in dirty clothes. We agreed it was easier as part of a team and with others to share the load, but those stories also seemed like a counterpoint to ours – less about inadequate public sector supports for care and more about our own moral goodness.

Good, bad. Right, wrong.

I still remember one of the first Friday night chapel services I attended at L'Arche. I introduced myself to the chaplain after the service and threw in one of my trademark "Nicely done, big boy" comments to top it off. Without missing a beat, Martha, one of the L'Arche elite, *charged over* from the other side of the coat-room and said, "His name is Joseph. He is *married* to Rebecca. He has a *wife* and two children." By the tone of her voice, you would have thought she had caught me with my shirt off, trying to have sex with him. I can't remember how I responded, just that I felt put in my place. I thought maybe she'd misread the folksy, fun-lovin', working-class part I was playing – the fact that there was a tacky, Dolly Parton-esque quality to it. I also sensed there was a lot her and other long-time community members weren't picking up on, as they didn't show much interest in younger live-in assistants or bother to ask us about our lives pre-L'Arche. Mostly though, I took Martha's comment as another sign that I was being called to let up on the "Janna show," to instead commit to the humble work of listening and learning from others.

When new assistants were hired, we talked in team meetings about how we'd have to introduce them to ways of living ethically in community. I still remember a L'Arche leader explaining that L'Arche "teaches assistants how to love," as though we were empty vessels with nothing to offer. I flinched. I remembered that was something Paulo Freire had written about in *Pedagogy of the Oppressed* (1972). He argued that oppressing others involves positioning them as "empty vessels to be filled" (66) or as needing to be integrated. And, while Jean Vanier wrote that "to really care for the growth and freedom of other people means to sacrifice our own freedom" (2002, 31), Paulo Freire warned that "without freedom [the oppressed] cannot exist authentically" (32). *How could they have missed that?*

Part of what bound me to the work, I think, was reworking ways of doing it.

When it came to bathing, I took note that other assistants created a welcoming atmosphere – lighting candles, putting on classical music, and gently caressing core members as they supported with their personal routines. That didn't sit well with me as a six-foot-three woman and former college basketball player who loved super-efficient showers. "I wouldn't want anyone making a sacrament of me, mistaking my frame for Christ's," I had joked. I turned up my nose at others' overly wholesome, Disney princess-y approaches to care. I remember thinking it was a shame that adults with developmental disabilities almost exclusively interacted with staff who put on a false self or only pulled out certain kinds of wholesome or holy stories in their presence. It bothered me when I heard live-in assistants going for broke with a joke or a story at a party in a way that they wouldn't dare in the presence of the disabled. I had to wonder if they thought disabled people were a bit pathetic, in need of a fantasy land and finger paint.

While the caregiver relationship often stresses humility, self-denial, and self-sacrifice, I thought self-development and self-expression should be made higher priorities. I thought our best chance at something mutual or liberatory was to bring "the fullness and authenticity of the 'I' into relation" (Gill-Austern 1996, 313). On the one hand, I could see how some of the assistants I lived with were more constrained. As a white woman from Canada, I wasn't trying to hold down the job to send remittances home or to be able to apply for permanent residency. My "respectability" or "goodness" weren't in question. But although I recognized my own privilege and how different our situations were, I also felt like I was making a difference by modelling a more mutual way of relating. I believed in the work I was doing.

When it came to supporting with personal routines, I was glad to find music that core members and I both liked. I made a point to crack jokes and to bring myself into it. I particularly enjoyed hanging out with Holly, a woman I supported and hit it off with. We hit up music festivals and sipped virgin margaritas. It felt like we were finding ways out of the dominant narratives we had both been funnelled into.

After a few months of living in community, I was invited to share a reflection for Lent at our community's Friday night chapel service. It felt like a homecoming as I thought back to how I had shared my testimony in chapel in university and on spiritual retreats during my year of service in LA. I was glad to take to the pulpit. In my Lenten reflection, I led off with the opening line, "I've been to the well, all right." Throwing my historical self under the bus, I reflected on how self-centred I had been at stages in life when I had "been to the well" – showing up and stealing the spotlight but closed off to others. I shared how I'd been to the well – armed with theories, with textbooks, and with certainty, or with a drink in hand or a joke to crack, but without being as open to what others were offering me. I also shared how, on occasion, I had been to the well, and I had "tasted the living water" – living fully in the moment, while allowing myself to be ministered to. I mentioned how I had been learning from my housemates, allowing myself to be transformed by the stories and people around me.

When I finished reading, I let out a deep exhale. I was glad to be coming home to myself, engaging in theological work in community. After the service, I was still basking in the glow of it, when Joseph, the chaplain, approached me to say that he thought it sounded *a bit* better when I read it than when he first read it over himself. Raising his eyebrows and half rolling his eyes, he elaborated that when he first read it, he wasn't sure *where* I was going with such a vulnerable reflection or *how* it was going to land. I thought maybe he was referring to the part about my drinking to cope, or maybe just to the parts where I was positioning myself as a person in my own right. Whatever it was, I felt ashamed or as though I had been caught with my shirt off, yet again. *Hadn't I received the memo about modesty and decorum?*

It wasn't long after that that a long-time assistant warned me that she had learned to keep things closer to the chest at L'Arche, that it wasn't a safe space for creative self-expression. "It's really not the kind of community where you want to make yourself vulnerable, especially not if you plan to stay long-term," she said. "It will just get used against you."

I registered her words on the one hand, but it also seemed more like she was sharing red flags about a shitty ex-boyfriend, while I was still in the honeymoon phase. Her advice had me wondering if maybe *she* was a bit paranoid, or how *she* could possibly think there wasn't space to bring oneself into the community, when spiritual thinkers like Jean Vanier or Henri Nouwen had used L'Arche as a homebase, writing their own books and making a name for themselves. Didn't she realize that they'd even made a point to compliment both my humour and humility in the job interview? That they saw something in me, and me in particular?

I was certain there was no better place for the gifts I wanted to bring forth.

For one of my assignments for the online program in pastoral studies, I wrote about my life as a live-in assistant and how much I was learning along the way. I was proud to share it with Martha, the woman who had been assigned as my "spiritual mentor." Although she had once corrected me for saying "big boy," it seemed like she was warming to me in our spiritual accompaniment sessions. I think she could see I was on a spiritual journey – that there was an intentionality to it. I also thought maybe she had something to offer; I liked that she'd taken an alternative life path, living out a consecrated, contemplative life. In that meeting in Martha's apartment, as I read my assignment to her, I couldn't help but think that I was right where I needed to be, living out my faith in the flesh. Similar to the Lenten reflection, the piece I wrote for the assignment was about how much I was learning in conversation and community with others. I smiled as I read it aloud to her, looking up when I finished.

"Hmm," Martha said, unimpressed. She didn't exactly jolt her head back, but she did advise me that I should rewrite it. The entire piece. The whole thing. Instead of putting in insights that *I* came up with, I should instead show that it was *people with disabilities* that helped me come to those insights – that I was following *their* lead. "It just comes off a bit self-indulgent," she said.

And for whatever reason, something snapped. I didn't feel like I had been caught with my shirt off or that I should have been listening or learning or caring for others *more*. At that point, I had already spent several months working sixty hours a week providing direct daily care – split shifts, mornings and evenings, with next to no time to myself. It wasn't that I hadn't been listening or learning or caring *enough*. It also wasn't lost on me that Martha and the other higher-ups lived out and with space to themselves in their own homes or apartments, while I had been tucking myself into that twin bed with my feet hanging off the end of it.

"Um, aw, you know," I said to Martha. I stuttered to try to get a little sentence together, something to counter her suggestion that I should put my meaning-making self to bed. "I, uh, I'm of course invested in listening and learning from others, I can't deny that, but I, uh, you know, also think maybe I'm being called to contribute in my own right," I said to Martha. "*I, uh* – I think maybe I'm an artist," I offered, spitting out the sentence.

"Artist?" Martha scoffed, choking on the word. I think maybe she was expecting me to reposition myself in relation to her ideals. To lay down a moral card or at least give a bit of a shuffle to show that was my intent. "Hmm," Martha said again. From there, she responded by saying that if I was to *truly* surrender to community life – to open myself up to listening and learning from people with disabilities – that my desire to be an artist would dissipate. "That desire to feel heard or to be seen is about your childhood wounds or something deeper," she said. "God's love should be enough to stake your whole life on; it should be enough for you. *Community* should be enough for you."

I can't remember how I responded to that, or whether I eased up on trying to create space for myself in that conversation. I just remember it sinking in how much the institutional structures of community life had been rubbing me the wrong way. Every word out of Martha's mouth, and the mouths of other leaders, all seemed code for "give more." *Give more and keep your goddamn mouth shut.*

Jacques Derrida wrote about the impossibility of hospitality, the impossibility of a host ever forfeiting his power enough for a guest to truly make herself at home. In his book *Deconstruction in a Nutshell*, John Caputo (1997) writes, "When the host says to the guest, 'Make yourself at home,' this is a self-limiting invitation. 'Make yourself at home' means: please feel at home, act as if you were at home, but, remember, that is not true, this is not your home but mine, and you are expected to respect my property" (111).

Martha acted like L'Arche was her property. Like I was her property. I wish I could say that I took my conversation with her as a sign to get out or draw some hard distance, but, in a weird way, it bound me further to the work. I felt even more compelled to speak up, an even greater sense of moral responsibility. Not only did I feel responsible for building relationships with the people we supported in a unique and interesting way, but she had also awakened my inner critic. The analyst. The shit disturber. The one who'd been carrying the notebook.

Care Junkie Diaries

As a live-in caregiver, I wrote pages and pages in my "Care Junkie Diaries." I couldn't help noticing details to take a stand against, aspects of the organization's structure that were a little off. I felt like I was on a mission to stand up for myself and my co-workers, to call attention to power dynamics that weren't being considered.

Housemates and I made stovetop popcorn and sipped wine, as we found a language to talk about things, critiquing the conditions of our labour. Framing it not just as "sharing life" but as skilled work to support people with complex needs was a big deal; so was naming the ways the organization devalued the work of care. I remember commenting that L'Arche felt like a summer camp where the meanings had already been made and we were just supposed to show up and play the part of camp counsellors. It was a friend who suggested we were more like servants on *Downton Abbey*. She wondered if it would have been a more interesting place to live when the community first opened, if assistants would have had a hand in helping to shape things. I also wondered if it would have been easier to work as an assistant in another L'Arche home, like the one Philip lived in, where they took turns watching TV shows that assistants liked. While I had initially liked that we let the core members call the shots in their own home, I was sick of watching *Friends*, *The Wiggles*, or *Sharon, Lois & Bram*.

Some of our critiques felt subversive. We joked about getting our tubes tied or sourcing out abortions, noting that to reproduce the community we could not reproduce ourselves. I don't think any of us had read anything about the controlling of women's reproductive labour under capitalism, but perhaps we were picking up on it, or at least paying enough attention to notice that assistants who got pregnant moved back home with their parents. I can also remember joking to friends about how invitations to "listen and learn from the most vulnerable among us" were starting to sound similar to the idea that women are obliged to let their husbands fuck them. I'll admit, at times we pushed it too far when reaching for metaphors to describe how denigrating the experience was, how violated we felt. I think we were trying to understand what was so hard about it.

I questioned the organization's assumption that the way society structures a person's worth or non-worth is *only* about disability, as though by virtue of not having intellectual disabilities, assistants were coming from places of power. I thought maybe it would have been easier to serve others if we had the cultural resources, power, prestige, and elite family lineage of L'Arche founder Jean Vanier, whose father was a Canadian governor general. I even wrote a poem about it (Payne 2013). In it, I included a comment from Vanier himself, who had once said, "It's not anyone who can become a leader. You've got to have formation." I questioned in the poem if Vanier had been hinting at his cultural, social, and political resources, his PhD, his wealthy family lineage, and his countless publications and television appearances. Was that the "formation" he meant? Was that how you speak for God?

Years later when I re-read the poem, I was surprised by how sociological I was in my thinking. I reflected in the poem on the material conditions needed to live a moral life, how having eight hundred bucks in your wallet helps the cause. I also hit on the power dynamics at play, getting at how care work is assigned, perceived, and valued along gendered and classed lines, how some get more points for doing what others are expected to do for free or without any thanks. "Remember, ladies, it's not anyone who can become a leader," I wrote, referencing Vanier's elite masculinity.

Some assistants and I were critical of how L'Arche relied on racialized immigrant women who worked overnight shifts and were referred to as "night ladies." One older immigrant woman of colour had worked overnights in the home I was in, sleeping on the couch for twenty years. Speaking with some co-workers at the time, we wondered if she was tired of dozens of young adults passing through on the way to something better. Did she think we were too smug? We worried about how she was pit against *us*, occasionally mentioning how organizational structures played a role. The job title "night lady" erased the work and skill involved. She was excluded from team meetings – cut off from making meanings or decisions. Brochures about community life didn't mention her or any of the other "night ladies" who were essential to the running of the homes and the community. Older Black women were not treated as subjects in their own right.

At L'Arche, I couldn't help but critique how elite, well-educated spiritual leaders like Martha, who lived out (mostly in their own private homes), were set apart from the "night ladies" and from young live-in workers, including working-class women and racialized migrant workers without permanent residency status. L'Arche leaders with master of divinity degrees coached us on submissiveness, coaxed us to forfeit our power, and cued us to say that we got more than we gave. They treated us like stage props in their performance of community. It was the leaders who wrote books and sermons, while the help worked in bathrooms, bedrooms, and kitchens. I don't remember anyone in a position of power talking about how live-in workers can be susceptible to labour exploitation or to physical and psychological harms. They didn't talk about care as labour or about the importance of supporting permanent residency status for all migrant care workers – many of whom were employed by the organization.

At a community-wide meeting for live-in assistants, a middle manager gave a speech to encourage us to listen and learn from disabled residents who were the true artists, visionaries, and teachers. He said the *only* job for assistants is to listen, learn, observe, and open ourselves to others. I raised my hand to ask how much time he thought should go by before we'd be allowed to speak or teach. "One or two years?" I asked, "A decade?" I loved seeing him, at least performatively, take pause. It was fun coming up from behind.

That was around the time that I printed out and distributed handouts, challenging the proposed L'Arche "servant leadership model" that emphasized the importance of serving others as a way to "lead." To me, "serving to lead" didn't seem like the message that live-in assistants, who were *already* serving for sixty hours a week, most needed to hear. On the handout, I included excerpts from Deborah Eicher-Catt's (2005) article on the myth of servant leadership, in which she talks about how the model serves the interests of a chosen few – sustaining oppressive practices and power imbalances, while binding others to the project. She wasn't talking about L'Arche in particular but her insights rang true. I printed twenty or so handouts, passing them around to other live-in assistants. I also cheered to read Eicher-Catt's point that true ethical leaders are "visionary meaning-makers not merely meaning re-producers" (24), as I thought that described me and some of my care work cronies perfectly. I also thought taking responsibility wasn't just about providing direct care for others but about speaking out against injustices.

It was a friend and fellow live-in assistant who sent me the article about the "myth of servant leadership" (Eicher-Catt 2005) and who introduced me to a language for thinking about the political economy of care. She took issue with the fact that L'Arche was undercutting other social service agencies, paying us in moral wages instead of real ones. She also said the "problem" wasn't just the organization or the middle managers keeping us in line, but the way the government was "wiping its hands" of care. One example of this – which I came across while I was an assistant – was in Tim Kearney's book *A Prophetic Cry* (2000), which features an interview with Therese Vanier (Jean's sister), who co-founded L'Arche UK. In the interview, Therese mentions how L'Arche UK lob-bied against statutory authorities, contested legal labour requirements, and secured the right to pay live-in assistants less than minimum wage within L'Arche UK. As she said, "That is important, it made it possible for us to continue. My goodness, if we hadn't won that battle, I don't know what we would have done. We would have either become illegal or we would have had to lose half our assistants" (Kearney 2000, 184). When I first read her remarks, I was struck by how limited her imagination for care was. Her remarks also speak to the role of the state in outsourcing care to charitable organizations like L'Arche, without ensuring adequate regulations or worker protections. I mean, my goodness, if they hadn't been able to exploit assistants, where would they be? My goodness!

The history of L'Arche is also flawed in that way. When Jean Vanier founded L'Arche in France in 1964, he witnessed the abysmal treatment of disabled people in large-scale institutions, and instead of calling on the state to advocate for the closure of those institutions or for dramati-cally investing in and improving the lives of people living and working in them, he invited a couple disabled guys to move out of the institution and bunk in with him. His project was not about transforming the sys-tem. It was a scheme that let the state off the hook, with moral helpers relegated to positions of feminine servitude.

I took note of details like that at L'Arche, carrying my journal from room to room. I must have filled a dozen journals – my little care junkie archive. I also wrote poems about mopping up the messes that bodies make and shouldering the weight of an unjust system. I wrote most afternoons, filling pages with rants and one-liners to process the experience. My poems were all pretty heavy-handed, with titles like "The Psychological Cost of Learning to Care," "Au Pair: One Who Toils in Exchange for a Twin Bed," and "Explanation for Termination of Employment." I worked hard on the craft, writing and editing and drinking to cope. It meant a lot to publish some of my poetry. I liked having a bit of an audience or a public life as much as I liked using art as a form of resistance. And when I say that I drank, I mean that I *drank*. Having a few too many a few nights a week helped to take the edge off. It gave me a way to bring out my inner artist or entertainer. In the company of fellow live-in assistants, drink in hand, I felt like I could claim space, without worrying about someone prompting me to re-centre the needs of those deemed most worthy.

And, *yeah*, I'll admit – it was exhausting to keep waking up hung over and to keep caring and cooking and cleaning and smiling, on top of all the work to process and problematize things. The pressure I put on myself to connect with core members in an authentic way, combined with the work I was doing to critique the workings of the institution, was a heavy load.

Turned In

After a couple of years, I found it hard to giggle at toilets clogged with washcloths or to respond to the same questions again and again. When's breakfast? Is breakfast ready? Did you wash my clothes? Are they in my room? Who's driving me this morning? Can you grab my jacket? Can you – ? Did you – ? Will you – ? It was hard to constantly be in the presence of people so incredibly turned in on their own needs – unable to see outside of them.

I felt like I was putting on a show that I didn't feel part of, saying what needed to be said, watching the clock, running on fumes. I was exhausted from constantly being "on," constantly of service, and constantly having my psychological space invaded. I started taking breaks in the bathroom to get away from the people I supported. I rushed through routines, watched the clock. I painted on a fake smile, poured myself a few too many drinks. I can remember yelling at Shelly, a non-verbal woman with autism – begging her to stop screaming for five minutes so that I could think. I was sick of spoon-feeding her applesauce or jumping up to meet her every need. I was sick of her stiffening her body when we tried to lift her from the floor to her wheelchair. Once, when I tried to lift her by myself when another assistant was helping someone in the shower, she hardened her body, and I thought I had pinched a nerve in my back. "Jesus Christ, Shelly," I yelled, as she dropped to the floor.

At a United Church dinner with fifty or so people crammed into a basement, I can remember swearing under my breath as I helped fill plates for three of the people I supported, as I ran to get a towel to clean up a juice spill, and as I helped to train a new live-in caregiver. I escorted a woman to the bathroom to change her wet brief, only to come back to see Shelly had rolled up to the buffet, putting her hands in two dishes at the same time. *Oh, for fuck's sake.* In some ways, this was an average outing or nothing out of the ordinary, but things felt heavier and just so futile. When it was time to leave, I told one of the church volunteers that there was urine all over one of the chairs at our table. By that point, there was no making things look natural or fun. There was no batting my little eyelashes to ask where the paper towel and cleaning spray were so I could just clean up the little wee spill myself. "Yep. Urine on that chair over there," I said.

I had *nothing* left to give.

I could hardly be bothered to collect my moral wages.

At Starbucks or the grocery store or wherever we happened to be, when women bolted over to express that they couldn't do my job – that I must be an angel – I resisted the urge to tell them to *fuck right off.* I used to delight in comments like that, smiling as I mentioned the people I supported were the angels for putting up with me, but I could no longer play my little part. I think part of the problem was that I started noticing the genre conventions. It was always a certain type of well-dressed, wealthy, white woman. A designer handbag. A pep in her step. A tinge of condescension in her voice, as she called me "honey" or "sweetie" and ever so subtly hinted that she'd always been drawn to high-status work, that she wasn't anybody's little pet. I'm sure I mumbled a quick "thanks," but even that was a break in character. I could no longer pretend that I got more than I gave or that caring required more skill and effort from the core members than it did from me.

Projecting onto the people that I supported, I figured they were in as much pain as I was – as dependent and powerless as I felt. It was hard to see core members herded around in ten-passenger vans and sitting at tables set for a crowd, with no space for intimacy or independence. It was hard to see a core member break down in tears after a massage, as I wondered if it was the first time he'd been touched in years. It seemed like everyone was starving for something more, people with and without disabilities alike. I don't think I imagined that.

Daddy Loves You

At my limits, I lost my sense of humour and, to my shame, developed disgust towards some of the people I supported. It was a horrible, life-altering experience. I felt ableist just being there. Everything about one woman I supported started to repulse me. *Shelly.* It seemed she continually screamed from a place of pain, that she couldn't look up to acknowledge us. She was the one who clogged the toilet with wash-cloths and who occasionally stiffened her body when we tried to pick her up. When assistants would sit down on the couch after a long day, Shelly would wedge herself between our legs to sit with her back to us, signalling that she wanted us to give her a massage.

After a while, I had a visceral reaction every time I saw her. I think it was my body trying to get my attention, sending me signals to stay away from her. Some care workers develop autoimmune diseases; I developed disgust. A self-preservation tactic for powerless women. A warning to get the hell out. I flinched when she entered the room, found it painful to be in her presence.

A fellow assistant thought that maybe the reason Shelly pushed our nerves so much was that she was constantly trying to re-enact her old traumas, push us and push us to see whether we'd abuse her like she had been in the past. It was just a theory, what did she know, but I cried when she said it. There was something that seemed so true about that and about how hard we were being tested.

When Shelly's parents came to dinner for her birthday, I sat across from them, secretly thinking about how much I despised their daughter. "I can just tell who our daughter likes and doesn't like," her dad said. I knew he was talking about me – that she used to like me but didn't anymore. *Daddy's sixth sense.*

I debated asking him whether she'd been sexually abused by someone as a child, if that's why she grinds her pelvis against the floor, masturbating in front of everyone all the time. I also considered asking why he'd thrown her in an institution if he was such a "great dad." *What's that you said there, big guy? You talk a big game, but found it difficult too?*

I mean, I kept my mouth shut, took my little licking. But I could not get over such a cruel side of myself raging under the surface. I was angry all the time. *Angry,* angry. A raw, powerless loathing. It wasn't just a little blip of anger, but the kind of anger that's the response to the deprivation of basic needs.

"Shelly, you know your daddy loves you, right?" the dad said to her. *Oh, how the tides had turned.*

Years later, my friend Catherine said that revulsion hinges on a quality of enslavement. "The revulsion you experienced speaks to the obscenity of the set up," she said. "It's what L'Arche was creating. *They* did that. They did that to you and to other women. They lured idealistic young women in from around the world, turned them into *that*."

"Yeah, it was a perversion of power, for sure," I said to my friend. The word *enslavement* seemed to fit too.

I remember when my L'Arche housemates sang "Happy Birthday" to me. It shouldn't have been a big deal. They were trying. But for whatever reason, my disillusionment with my life as a care worker sunk in with each line of the song. "Happy birthday, dear Janna, happy birthday to you." It's hard to describe the violation that I perceived, hearing my name sung aloud in a caring way in a context in which I felt so radically uncared for. It was painful to be in a space where I couldn't exist in any real way, where I wasn't known in my own right. As Alice Notley (1998a) writes in one of her poems, "for two years, there's no me here" (39). I didn't feel like myself or like whoever they were singing to was someone I even knew. I resonated with Jeanette Winterson (2011), who writes, "I was not being myself, but I didn't know how to be myself there. I hid the self that I was and had no persona to put in its place" (135).

I'll admit those conditions had not been conducive to life. Maybe I had been morally enslaved. Not my real self. No "me" there. When I think of Shelly, I can't help but think of how we were positioned as servants in relation to her. The philosophy of L'Arche encouraged our limitless trust. We were to turn towards the disabled, sacrifice our own needs, receive the "gift" of their presence. *And who were we to say no or to set limits? Wasn't that why we had moved in, to turn towards the vulnerable other? To fall to our knees?*

Similar to Peace Corps volunteers in Rebecca Schein's (2008) study, serving others in the context I was in didn't lead to "the reconstitution of a self that has been tried and stretched" (184), but to an experience of "incoherence, incommensurability, and disjuncture" (185). I have never felt so small and fragile, so disconnected from myself. And, although I had initially liked the "experiment" in being made small, after a while it didn't feel like an experiment. I felt sick thinking that I'd been deprived to that extent, that society thought that lowly of me.

Escape Velocity

At L'Arche, I can remember talking about Mary Oliver's poetry with a fellow live-in care worker. We both wondered what we should do with our "wild and precious" lives (Oliver 1992, 94). We also cheered at Oliver's advice in "Wild Geese" that you shouldn't have to "walk on your knees" to feel worthy (1992, 101). Oliver's words felt like a reprieve, although neither of us thought it was as straightforward as it sounded in the poem. We couldn't help but think about the soiled sheets and unattended needs that would be left in our wake. We commented that the people that we supported wouldn't be able to get out of bed, that we'd be screwing over our co-workers, and that it wasn't as easy as closing up shop or letting the "soft animal" of our bodies love what it loves (Oliver 1992, 101). Just as unsettling, I think, was the moral dilemma and anticipated loss of "goodness" that would follow. With how we were set up, "leaving" or "just quitting" would also mean erasing our sense of selves and self-expectations.

As I look back now, I can hardly put into words how much was getting in the way of me simply resigning. Nor can I put to words how much I wanted out.

I wanted more than a small room with a twin bed and three hours off in the afternoons between shifts. I wanted time to myself, space to write and to think. I remember that my impulse to leave hit when a professor encouraged me to go back to school and when I visited a friend at grad school and stayed up all night talking about ideas. It hit when I saw a guy grading papers in a café and when I overheard a young family planning a pool party. I too wanted something of my own. It also hit when I walked empty-handed through IKEA while a friend sourced out stuff for her new apartment. With every tea towel and trinket she put in her cart, I had a strong urge to leave.

In an essay entitled "Nesting," I wrote about how I was craving freedom for myself as a live-in assistant: "Like a robin hoarding twigs, string, and hair, looking for a safe, quiet place to settle in, I am nesting" (Payne 2012, 28). It wasn't that I wanted to be a mommy or a homeowner, but I craved time and space to myself after years of delivering everything I had to others. I wanted space for intimacy and time to write.

Pushed past my limits, I went into a middle manager's office to express how burnt out I was and to ask to decrease my hours and decrease my pay. "I, uh, I know I only have a couple months left here before grad school anyway, but is there any way possible, by any chance, and if we could at all figure it out on the schedule, that I could have an extra day off each week, with reduced pay? I am really struggling ..." My hands shook as I made my request; I knew it was a vulnerable one.

Caught off guard, Esther, another one of the L'Arche elite, smirked and giggled. I couldn't believe she giggled, raising her hand to cover her mouth as though she was embarrassed or playing coy. From there, she denied my request. She said that if I was going to live there, I needed to work my full hours. I mean, I wasn't thinking straight, could hardly make eye contact with the people I supported, and she still wanted to milk just a bit more out of me.

When I myself needed care, there was none to be found. No care for the caregiver. "No thanks, no kiss my ass, nothing," as my mom would say.

I blamed Esther. I blamed the organization. I blamed the state.

Night after night, I blamed myself. At the limits of care, I felt an immense sense of shame. How could I have been so stupid? How could I have gotten myself into such a mess? How could I have disregarded my needs and my desires to that extent? How fucked up was that? How fucked up am I?

I thought of my younger sister who worked as a marketing manager at a bank and had bought her first home at age twenty-three around the time I started at the group home. I also thought of friends from high school and university who had chased domestic bliss – full-speed, just gunning. I had announced to them and to the whole damn world that I was carving out an unconventional counter path – going after the good life story. And now what? Admit to them and to myself how pathetic it all was? Admit that I couldn't even recognize myself in the mirror? That I had stayed to the point of developing disgust, morphing into the worker no one wants? *"Yep! You know me! I always said I'd go after the good life story! Get a load of this one ..."*

I also have to remember now that I got out. I escaped.

Friends helped to pull me out and to process along the way. I still remember my friend Kim encouraging me to put my own ideas before the petty needs of others. It sounded blasphemous when she said it, at least until she added, "Janna, can't you see you're starving? That you're an artist?" She encouraged me to make a run for it, to loosen the moral chains around my neck.

My house leader did the same. "Wouldn't you rather be an academic?" she asked. She pinpointed a desire that I had for myself but hadn't even begun to speak or admit out loud as a working-class kid from Peterborough, Ontario. She said that there were other moral paths for women to take, that good moral women leave L'Arche all the time. Her words meant a great deal to me. They seemed to offer whatever permission I felt I needed to release myself from what I had once seen as my vocation or something I wanted to commit to long-term. "I think you'd enjoy academia," she had said. "You remind of another woman who lived here; she's a professor now." I didn't expect to *ever* be taken care of by an institution, or that space would *ever* open up for me to feel heard or seen or supported in a way that I so deeply craved, but I must have thought about her comment hundreds of times. I also thought that maybe, at the very least, I could invest in myself – put my own ideas before the petty needs of others.

At a tarot card reading with some friends, I pulled the devil card and felt as though I was curling up in the arms of the woman doing the reading, as she talked about listening to our desires, pursuing pleasure, releasing the forces that constrain us. "The card might be a sign you are feeling restricted," she said to me, casually and without overthinking it. "And that might even be an understatement," I said, smiling and grateful.

I resigned from L'Arche in June of 2013 at age twenty-eight, with plans for Philip and me to get married in August, and for me to start grad school in Ottawa in the fall. We hadn't been rushing to get married so soon, but it was a way for us to stay together, for him to be able to apply for permanent residency status so we could live together in Canada. It was also a way for me to stop crawling around on my knees, as Oliver might advise.

Snapping Back

That summer, I borrowed money from my mom and dad and bunked in with them too, before Philip and I celebrated our marriage in Peterborough. That fall, I moved to Ottawa to start grad school at Carleton University.

From the start, academia felt like a reprieve, a retreat of sorts. I enjoyed writing in the margins of others' work, being in conversation with other powerhouse thinkers, and biking along the canal from my apartment in downtown Ottawa to the university. Studying Applied Linguistics and Discourse Studies in my master's was my way of taking baby steps. I didn't want to chase my wildest dreams by studying creative writing or women's studies or work and labour studies; I just wanted to abandon myself and my dreams a little less.

And, over time, I relaxed into things, dreaming a bit bigger along the way. As a master's student in applied linguistics, I ended up working with the only sociologist in the department. "Are you sure you're not a sociologist?" he asked me. "Have you thought about sociology for your PhD?" another professor in the department inquired. I think they noticed how much I was turning things over and interrogating dominant societal norms, and I had to agree.

I was thrilled when I was accepted to Carleton's Department of Sociology for my PhD. In my first semester there, a mentor encouraged me to undertake research motivated by my experience at L'Arche. She pointed out that there was a fire in my voice when I talked about care work – heat and energy around it. I'm grateful that she noticed that. I'm also grateful for another professor who kept suggesting that I really should talk to Susan Braedley, a feminist political economist and leading sociologist of care work. In one of our first meetings together with Susan as my PhD supervisor, she leaned in to ask, "So, what pisses you off?" I think she wanted to ensure I'd conduct research that mattered to me – something with stakes – but I don't think she could have predicted just how long my list of things that pissed me of about the topic was. She might have been better off asking me whether there was anything that *didn't* piss me off.

It was a slow crawl out of care work, a long old recovery process. Even years after resigning, something about the experience *still* had a hold. There was something about it that haunted me, kept me up at night, and at times could have me just reeling or snapping back at the slightest throwaway comment from an unsuspecting stranger or "keynote" speaker weighing in on the topic of care as they understood it.

At potlucks or dinner parties, at the first sign of someone valorizing, romanticizing, or mystifying caring for others, I'd interject with a counter story, as if sneaking up from behind to hit them with it. Someone would say something about a dementia village, about learning oh-so-much volunteering one day a week, or about how we need to listen and learn from the oldest or most disabled among us. Defensive and snapping back, I'd pelt out a story about getting it handed to me after wanting to be good as a care worker. Whipping out what felt like "my side" of the story, I warned others about the shit society throws at women, grieving for the woman who had to move into L'Arche when I moved out. "That organization made my life a living hell," I'd fume. I think I told it that way because I had to. It was the part of my story that I was trying to make sense of, or maybe even to validate.

When I first started engaging with feminist care scholarship, some works were bread for the journey, with lines I've replayed again and again, but I often felt like the questions I was most asking in my work and in life weren't ones being explored. I struggled to see my own experience reflected in the literature.

Painting with a broad brush, I didn't see myself in the dominant narrative. With my own back story, I couldn't help but roll my eyes as I read accounts of care workers who *loved* their jobs, wanted to care more, but just couldn't catch a break in the uncaring organizations where they worked. I had to wonder where those researchers had found so many fun-lovin' and well-meaning women who still had the stamina for it and "just wanted to care more." I scoffed at research that seemed to privilege the needs of people who rely on care by emphasizing an ethos of respect, championing person-centred care, or at times blaming care providers for their morally flawed approaches or for not making small talk or eye contact enough. I was sceptical of work that framed those who need care as more vulnerable, marginal, or morally worthy than care providers.

I found it hard to relate to scholarly accounts of care workers who were lumped together in an article or referred to not by name but by job title. Those women always seemed a bit pathetic. The researcher would indent a quote of something they said before elaborating on how they had internalized responsibility, exhibited zero-sum thinking, fallen into a neoliberal trap, or otherwise shit the bed. Women in caring roles weren't treated with the reverence I thought they deserved, as storytellers and meaning-makers in their own rights. I had to wonder where the stories like mine were. What about the art and artistry of it? What about care wrapped in moral coercion, martyrdom, guilt, and redemption? What about the power of anger or of pushing for something more? I longed to read something that registered the betrayal, the grief, the stories that are harder to tell.

I also had to face the fact that of course the questions I most longed to see explored weren't ones that others could explore for me. This wasn't because I'm some big hotshot, but because it's the job of memoirists to stay present to the contradictions of our lives or to the disruptive experiences that demand something from us. It was my story to tell and interrogate and I had to figure out how.

When I first started to discuss my hopes for my future research, a professor in my department responded to me, saying, "So you don't want to be a handmaiden?" His question played in the back of my mind as I designed my study. I certainly did not want to be a handmaiden, nor did I want to repress my voice or perspective, as I had as a care worker. And while some arts-based approaches see the researcher denying her own expertise, accommodating participants, or allowing *others* an outlet for *their* creativity, I wanted to take my seat as an artist and critic in my own right. This also felt crucial in a project that resists and challenges moral, gendered expectations for women to care or to only ever be of use or of service to others.

With a sense of urgency to the work I was doing, I couldn't have had more support from Susan, my friends, and other feminist scholars or former care workers. But it also seemed, at first, like I was met with resistance at every turn, or at least some turns.

The Flinch Factor

It's an understatement to say that my personal story about resigning from care work hit a nerve when I performed it as a part of a sociology conference in the United Kingdom. It was in the summer of 2018 in the second year of my PhD, five full years since I had resigned from L'Arche. The purpose of the conference was to showcase alternative, artistic works or polemic sociological interventions. Yes, "polemic." It seemed like the perfect venue to share my early thinking on the topic of "exiting" care work as I was working on the proposal for my doctoral research. I wanted to raise questions about how accounting for the perspectives of former care workers – those who reached their limits and no longer want to care for others – might shift sociological research and thinking on care that primarily centres the stories of well-meaning, hard-working carers who want to care more but just can't catch a break in the uncaring organizations where they work.

For my session, I performed a story reflecting on my experience living and working at L'Arche, before attempting to facilitate a discussion. I was eager to share my story, as I felt like I had done a lot of work to process and situate my experience, writing with compassion for myself and others. I was proud that I had moved beyond making an easy critique of management or the organization, and beyond blaming myself as an individual, to instead reflect on how I had been implicated. In the prose piece that I performed, I reminisced about moving into L'Arche, and shared that I had been drawn to care work to listen and learn from others and build community with disabled and non-disabled people alike. I mentioned that I had initially enjoyed spending time with the people that I supported, jogging alongside them on adaptive bike rides. "There was something there for me," I said.

From there, raging with pain and without a clear sense of what I was taking aim at, I shared about how devastating it had been, over time, when I lost my capacity to care, to even make eye contact with some of the people that I supported. I shared that I felt ashamed that I had stayed to the point of developing disgust towards some of the people I had supported. This was the part that felt like a breach, or like I was wading into lesser-travelled territory – telling part of the story that was hard for me to acknowledge or hard for me to know what do to with. I shared that it had been a slog to claw myself out of the work after several years in the field, as it felt like opting out of an ethical way of living – walking away from my "goodness." To close, I asked how we might cultivate conditions of care that honour care workers *and* people who need care alike, valuing and investing in care as a collective responsibility, not an individual, moral one. I asked whether a story like mine could help the cause.

As soon as I finished presenting, a full professor and world-renowned feminist sociologist – whom some at the conference tagged in photos with the caption #FeministIcon – raised her hand. I smiled over in her direction, anticipating she'd offer some of the recognition and support I craved. *Maybe a line to hold me? A comment about how I was registering these dymanics in a different, albeit compelling way?* Instead, she interjected with a critique of me and my story. *"You* escaped," she fumed. She said that the immigrant and racialized care workers who supported her mother were *trapped*. They couldn't leave; they had chains around their ankles. She emphasized the phrase as though slowly clapping out syllables to a toddler: *Chains. Around. Their. Ankles.* She said it like it was supposed to sting. She hinted that I was too privileged to be taking up space – that if my experience as a care worker had been bad enough, I would have died on the job. "The care workers worth learning from are the ones still working," she said.

After that, another full professor and feminist sociologist of care – a former nurse – interjected that I should have known that the care home where I worked was a dump when I first arrived and should have known well enough to set boundaries and keep myself safe. When she worked as a nurse and medical ward sister, she knew well enough to smoke a cigarette on her break and crack jokes about the people she supported. She knew well enough to hold them at a distance.

My voice squeaked as I responded saying that surely she could appreciate that care work is different in different contexts, that her job a few decades ago was different from mine. She nodded but fired back by critiquing my focus on my own experience – how my account made it sound like I was the only one producing value, like I was the only one with a perspective that mattered. She said that I didn't conduct a socio-logical analysis in the way that she would have, that I forgot to look at value production or at the financialization of care. As she spoke, I had to wonder if I perhaps would have written a dissertation like hers if I had resigned sooner or after my stint at the group home. Perhaps I too would have written something about how vulnerable help seekers are dismissed and denigrated by "expert" care workers, but it all seemed a little late for that. With her nose up and away from her mouth, the Former Nurse asked, "In what world could you have possibly felt pow-erless as a care worker?"

Whew. Their heavy-handed comments knocked the wind right out of me.

From there, a woman around my age raised her hand to mention that she resonated with my story – that she thought there was a lot of power in it. She said that she too had struggled to set boundaries at the social service agency where she worked, and that it had been a life experience that had been hard to process. I appreciated her courage in speaking up but could hardly register her words. I was too busy noticing the Feminist Icon gritting her teeth and flashing a restrained smile at me. I was too busy sitting in my shame.

There was something incredibly destabilizing about the experience. It was painful to feel so misunderstood and rejected. It was hard to make sense of what felt like such a profound lack of compassion or failure of the imagination. It was painful to have devoted so much energy to thinking about the topic, and to finally take the stage in such a momentous way – articulating something so close to home – only to be criticized. I think what I most wanted was to have my story witnessed or made real in that way, as a story that was part of a larger narrative – a story that mattered. But, even after four straight years of processing, I still felt like I had a busted story that didn't translate.

"What the hell was that?" a woman said to me in the bathroom afterwards, poking fun at the two profs who had critiqued me. We took turns trying to put a finger on why they had taken such a run at me. She wondered if reflexive accounts about care work, or at least the ones from care workers themselves, aren't supposed to circulate. I joked that perhaps they both thought they had the care sector by the balls – that they had it all figured it out, so it was awkward to entertain a perspective they hadn't considered. I also questioned if part of the problem was that I didn't fit into their stereotypical understandings of care workers as victims, caught up in relations of domination, with chains around their ankles. She said that she agreed with my point that the devaluation of care workers goes hand in hand with the devaluation of those who need care. She too was still struggling to understand why it had been so hard for her to set boundaries or say no. "I, um, guess it's not hard for all women, though?" I said, puzzled. "Yeah, if they know the trick to boundary setting, they should tell us," she said, laughing.

I laughed in the bathroom, but it was hard to keep up the comedy beyond that. I mostly felt raw and vulnerable, as I had expressed that I had suffered and they had responded by sharing emotionally charged, personal critiques of me and of how I had navigated things. I couldn't understand how two well-resourced profs – who had dedicated their careers to researching care and who had access to scholarly and professional discourses – were caught off guard to the point of critiquing a junior scholar personally and sharing their own memories to counter mine. Neither bothered to situate my story or to ask questions about the structures giving rise to it.

Their responses seemed to position me as smug, self-absorbed, and privileged, and to place blame on me for not having navigated the situation properly. The Feminist Icon wanted it on the record that my experience wasn't as bad as others, that I wasn't enough of a victim. The Former Nurse wanted it known that I was to blame or must have done something to deserve it. They both seemed to assign personal responsibility for structural injustices, playing their moral high cards along the way. "Honey, aren't you one of the happy-go-lucky feminist good girls?" they seemed to ask. The Feminist Icon took on a moral position in relation to "victims" who provide care. The Former Nurse took hers in speaking of my inability to provide "proper" care or "smoke and joke." They both maybe agreed that it was exploitation, but just not as bad as others' exploitation and my own fault.

Good, bad. Right, wrong.

Shame-spiralling, I too wondered why I hadn't known the care home that I worked at was a "dump" when I first started. Why hadn't I set boundaries, kept myself safe, or resigned from care work sooner when I had been so miserable? Why had I pursued such a stigmatized, devalued path to begin with? Why had I gotten stuck?

It was easy to get stuck in an individualized story, but I also found myself asking, if it had *just* been a job at a "dumpy" work site, wouldn't I be over it by now? Why hadn't smoking and joking seemed like options? Why did I feel like care still had a hold on me or like I was still "in" it? It hit me that I was researching and exploring a touchy subject, but that I didn't know where the edges were. I felt confused about the rules of the game. There was a flinch factor there, but what was it?

Conversations with friends, mentors, and my therapist helped me to process. "I swear to God – she actually suggested smoking and joking," I'd say, getting some mileage out of it. "I don't know how I provoked them," I said to my PhD supervisor, Susan. She didn't miss a beat in countering that *I* wasn't the problem. She suggested that it was provocative material, that the story itself was provocative, but that it wasn't *me* or me as a "type" of person who was provoking. She credited me for getting their attention, inviting them to consider a perspective they hadn't fully explored. She thought I must have hit on something. Similarly, my therapist suggested that people need to voice their traumas. She elaborated that, when people are triggered, they often respond by sharing raw, unprocessed emotions, or by making connections to their own histories, as the prots had. She suggested that my story had hit too closely to their own lives or fears. She didn't think it was me either, but that my story was touching fears.

Asking questions about how I had been hitting on something and touching fears helped me to engage and unpack in a different way. I felt like I was on a bit of a mission to learn more about the dominant conventions for speaking about care. When I first reflected on the backlash that I received, I suspected that my story hit a nerve when services for care are so thin and when people have real fears about who will care for them. It can be threatening to suggest that care has limits, or to hear from someone who doesn't want to provide care, when we rely on services and when being denied or refused care is such a threatening experience. With threadbare services, and with people's lives valued on the basis of age, ability, or health status, telling an earnest rip-roar of a story about walking off the job almost seems like a way of devaluing or neglecting those who need care. We need ready and willing good girls to care. We don't have time to talk about consent. As I've thought about it, I also wonder if part of the flinch factor was that it was hard to admit that, as care workers or would-be care workers, we as individuals may not be able to keep ourselves safe or set boundaries given the way care is organized. Perhaps my story was an uncomfortable reminder of how vulnerable we all are.

Fears about care? Threadbare services? Shared vulnerability? Check, check, check. It all sounded good as I said it fast, but another part of me wasn't sure. I think I wanted to get a handle on it or figure things out so I'd never suffer like that again. So I'd be smarter next time, wiser to it. I wanted control, a bit of "ego safety" or something to put my "self" back in place. That instinct to solve things kicked into overdrive, both in thinking about my struggles as a care worker and my struggles to translate my experience. I wanted to figure out what exactly would keep me safe or prevent me from feeling so small or vulnerable again.

But there was also so much that was so hard to say, so much uncertainty that I seemed to have to live with, so much that seemed hard to pin down. It was such a disruptively disorienting experience to hit my limits as a care worker, and then such a disruptively disorienting experience to try to talk about it, and both of those processes seemed to invite my full attention, demanding that I stick with things a bit longer.

This book takes up the challenge. It's an elegy to my moral, feminine ambition, a way of refusing to abandon myself. It's the result of a feminist sociological analysis that examined dominant institutional structures and meanings of gendered care work in contemporary life. The next chapter is an overview of the project, with the outline of the book at the end of it. I will share my motivations for the study and the research design that involved life history research with women positioned differently in Ontario's caring economy. I'll examine women's lives as a serious subject. I'll open things up, turn things over, *seek*.

Chapter Two

Towards a Counter Politics of Care

"What about the limits of care?" is a question that I asked again and again, when I first initiated my research to learn from women's stories of reaching their limits and stepping back from paid or unpaid care work roles. I was motivated to critically reflect on what makes care hard to leave. I wanted to start "at the limits," tracing out from there. The project has shifted and twisted over time, with me coming to see things in new ways and asking different questions along the way. This book presents key takeaways from the research that I conducted, with insights that (1) reveal care's inequitable gender organization; (2) identify and challenge dominant tropes, assumptions, or expectations at play; and (3) open possibilities for more equitable, emancipatory futures.

As explored in chapter 1, my desire to examine the limits of care was motivated by my own hard-won experiences. After several years of working in social services, I experienced hitting my limits as a painful crisis of self. To resign from care work seemed like an erasure of self, but to stay didn't seem possible either. I was too physically and emotionally exhausted to continue caring for others, but too attached to the idea of myself as a moral person to simply walk away. I eventually quit, but even long after I resigned from care work, I still felt as though I was "in" it. I was still hung up on how I had gotten "stuck" and still preoccupied with questions about what I owed others. It was disillusioning not to be able to live up to the ideals I had aspired to. Not only did I struggle as a care worker, but I also struggled, long after, to put a name to what felt like an invisible framework that had kept me hooked. Care *still* had a hold. Some of the women I interviewed in my research also related to this.

Carrie reached the limits of care. I didn't observe it; she told me about it as we sat holed up in the back of a coffee shop for a few hours straight. She said that she woke up on the floor of a Walmart, with strangers tapping her shoulders telling her she had passed out. As she said, "I was disassociating *really*, really bad, like, going to get groceries at Walmart and waking up with strangers in my face, 'Are you okay?'" It was around 2010, and she was in her early thirties at the time. She said that she had been working long, full weeks at a shelter on top of raising two kids and going to university full-time. She also described a slew of other care responsibilities across her life from helping to raise her siblings, babysitting to buy family groceries, entering paid care work in social services, raising her kids, supporting extended family, and supporting parents at risk of having their children taken away. Her story spoke to inadequate public-sector supports for care, to the early socialization of girls into caring roles, and to experiences of disadvantage and precariousness that she had been vulnerable to as an Indigenous woman.

It stood out to me that Carrie, who was born in the 1980s, talked about paid and unpaid work in different contexts in Ontario's care economy. Her account spoke to how, in the Canadian province of Ontario, care work has increasingly been downloaded from the state onto individuals – shifting care provision from a collective, public responsibility to an individual, private one (Armstrong 2023). It's not just individual paid workers who are tasked with "picking up the slack" or working through breaks to compensate for organizational or systemic issues, but unpaid family carers are also feeling the weight of the lack of investment in care in their households and communities (Addati et al. 2018; Armstrong 2023). Women in particular face unfair, heavy care workloads with inequitable gendered and racialized divisions of labour (Prentice and Armstrong 2021; Thomas 2023). Globally, the care sector is stratified along lines of gender, race, class, and immigration status, with hierarchies between women (Cranford 2020) and with transnational care circuits unevenly distributing resources and over-relying on racialized and immigrant care workers (Gottfried and Chun 2018). Care tasks and responsibilities fall to women; so too do the risks, costs, and consequences. There are ever-increasing stories of "care crises," "care deficits" (Fraser 2016), and gender and intersectional inequities (Das Gupta 2020; Lightman 2022; Syed 2020), and Carrie told a powerful one.

At the limits of care, Carrie remembered thinking, "I'm not – I don't have – I'm too burnt out for that. I know that about myself." Depressed and sleep-deprived with back pain that she thought was sciatica, she joked that she had been like an "eyeball vampire," tired, pale, and crying all the time. "So *that* was the breaking point," Carrie said. "I said 'no' to shifts for three weeks, and after that, I never worked there ever again." As Carrie and I spoke, I *revelled* in the "get a load of this" way she told her story. Laughing as she spoke, Carrie said, "It was almost like waking up after being in a cult, like I finally snapped the hypnosis, or whatever kind of veil I'd been living under." "*Oh. My. Gosh,*" I roared, laughing. I cheered at the words "cult," "hypnosis," and "veil." Our conversation felt like a shared creative experience. We were touching on something, opening to possibilities. I can't express how much I had needed that – how hungry I was to learn from her and others.

As I sat across from Carrie, I cheered at what seemed like a hard-won story of care resistance. It comforted me to think she had escaped the grip of care, walking off the job once and for all. Yet, as I read and re-read her story, and thought about my own, I was struck by how care *still* had a hold. "And it's this constant measuring and reflecting," Carrie said. "Even now, I'm still unravelling the ways where I respond to others before myself." She described ongoing work to "get out from under caring for others" that went beyond simply resigning from one paid work position. Her problem wasn't simply a matter of work/organizational conditions on the clock or in a particular care setting; renegotiating care responsibilities wasn't as simple as saying no to shifts or stepping back. She was *still* rethinking her beliefs, sense of self, and relationships with others. Her story, like my own and those of others, invited a nuanced analysis of how exactly care has a hold.

And when I say "care," I mean both care as work and care as a concept. In investigating care as work, I follow Evelyn Nakano Glenn (2010), who notes that care work involves a range of activities related to sustaining others, such as providing direct (physical and emotional) care for a person, maintaining physical surroundings, and fostering or maintaining relationships and networks (see also Black 2020). Care work can be defined more broadly as social reproduction, or the maintenance and continuation of existing social relations, which includes the paid and unpaid, daily and generational work of maintaining and reproducing human life, including by reproducing the workforce for capital (Braedley and Luxton 2021; see also Braedley et al. 2021).

Further, beyond a focus on the work involved, I apply a feminist rhetorical approach to examine shifting conceptions of care. With such a focus, I follow and engage with the work of narrative researchers who examine people's co-constituted stories of caring as a way to understand or learn about context and meaning (Doucet 2006; Funk 2015; Luttrell 2013, 2020; Stacey 2005, 2011). Concepts of care can be thought of as situated in relational sites and as having relational lives; they are embedded, brought about and remade through "histories, networks, and narratives" (Somers 2008, 209). Concepts not only "describe social life" but "are also active forces shaping it" (Fraser and Gordon 1994, 310). In my research, looking both at care as work *and* at shifting conceptions of care that are remade in context helps to answer my questions about why inequitable care relationships can be hard to leave and even hard to talk about, and how things can be otherwise.

Focusing Questions

As I explored in chapter 1, I tried to be a selfless, caring woman, but the effort nearly dissolved me. At the same time, I value care. I think it is necessary to human existence, to our relationships, and to addressing many of society's biggest challenges. I think it's worth asking: How can we have care security for children, older people, and those who are sick, frail, disabled, or otherwise in need of support *without women's endless, selfless caring and without such debilitating conditions*? When I designed my research, I thought that other women might have ideas. I had to ask: What stories do women tell about care that might disrupt or challenge conventional accounts of women's loving selflessness, endless patience, and intuitive abilities in caring? How might learning from their counter stories have the potential to reveal how gendered care work is organized and imagined, transforming how we think about ourselves and our relationships?

In exploring these questions, I orient to "gender as a central aspect of the social relations of care, and care as a central aspect of inequitable gender relations" (Armstrong and Braedley 2013, 19). I draw inspiration from Susan Braedley (2013), who writes that "historical relations of sex/gender get into us, shaping our sense of who we are, how we must be and what is possible, desirable, or necessary to us" (66). She points to relations that are about more than the work we do on the clock. Her insights connect well with those of Evelyn Nakano Glenn (2010), who writes, "Achieving the kinds of changes needed to produce a society that values caring will require *transforming the ways we think about ourselves*, our relationships with others, the family, civil society, the state, and the political economy" (201, emphasis added).

In this book, I attend to relations that "get into us" and to "the ways we think about ourselves" as critically important to the story of women and care. I examine gendered power relations, as they shape our ideas and sense of selves *and as we reshape them.*

Investigating gender relations is important, as they are "dominant in shaping who needs care and who provides it" (Braedley 2013, 59). With global divisions of labour, women are assigned to care work, while men are assigned to productive work (Braedley 2013; Luxton 1980). An example of this is how care work is often seen as incompatible with elite, white forms of masculinity: "Lives most consistent with elite masculinities will have more choices to recreate, while those lives most consistent with subordinated and oppressed groups will experience more conscription to care" (Braedley 2013, 61). Yet, as Braedley (2013) observes, care work is not just "gendered" because it's women who are providing it, but because of its organization through gendered power relations at different levels of social organization. These gendered power relations include symbolic and structural relations, organizational and institutional relations, and everyday micro, intimate relations, which can include self/other relationships or relationships to our sense of selves (Connell 2002, 2005, 2012b; see also King and Cronin 2013; Storm et al. 2017).

You'll notice in this book that when I analyse the stories of Carrie and other women, I make links to gendered power relations at these different levels of social organization. These "levels" are of course interconnected, intersecting, and difficult to distinguish. The global political economy is produced through the everyday practices of people and groups (Onuki 2011), just as "micro-level social relationships play a part in contesting or reproducing power at the level of social structures" (Brickell 2003, 165). A goal as the book moves along is to consider both how women's lives are shaped and constrained, as well as how they agentively negotiate their circumstances and contribute to shifting and reshaping gender relations through their practices (see Connell 2012).

Throughout this book, you'll see me orienting to women as storytellers and meaning-makers with insights to offer (see Basting 2020; Chivers and Kriebernegg 2017). I take seriously that, long before speaking to me, the women who contributed to my project were already engaged in critical dialogue and debate, and already engaged in work to creatively break down and reconstruct alternative understandings in the context of their lives (see Chivers and Kriebernegg 2017; Eicher-Catt 2005; Luttrell 2020). I've learned a lot from them and have written this book to pass on some of those insights.

As a feminist sociologist, I've also worked hard to tease out and contextualize women's stories – of reaching their limits, crossing ethical lines, and stepping back from paid or unpaid care work roles. These can be thought of as counter stories in that they "run counter to dominant cultural storylines about care giving and care receiving" (Luttrell 2013, 295). They are "stories people tell and live which offer resistance, either implicitly or explicitly to dominant cultural narratives" (Andrews 2004, 1). Such stories are ever-present but clash with dominant discourses. They don't fit the imaginary or make sense in light of broader social patterns that assign care to some women indefinitely or without adequate options to set limits or step back.

When it comes to counter stories of leaving in particular, I note that prior scholarship or public policy conversations have not adequately reflected on withdrawing from care or consulted former carers to learn from their insights. Rachel Herron and colleagues (2019) implicitly speak to the importance of this in their study of family carers supporting people with dementia, saying, "Carer information, support groups, and the system of long-term care need to make visible the opportunity to exit the caring role by naming and discussing when and how to stop providing care" (477). For this to happen, learning from those who have stepped back is a critical step. Learning from "former" carers is also a timely area of focus, with the unprecedented number of paid workers who have exited the field in what some call a mass exodus (Gilchrist 2021) and with increasing stories of "granny dumping" or family members who are otherwise no longer able to provide care in households or communities (see Van Pevenage et al. 2020). Having shown in my own memoir how entrapping carers can be detrimental for all involved, I begin with the critical assumption that limit-setting is central to ensuring equitable conditions of work and care, and that care providers should be able to say no, set limits, or otherwise bound their work.

I will share more below about my emerging story-based approach, as it involved advancing and enacting what can be thought of as a "counter politics of care" approach. In addition to my use of auto-ethnographic memoir writing (presented in chapter 1), I conducted life history research informed by feminist political economy and feminist rhetorical approaches. Rather than using one method to support, add on to, or confirm the findings of another, my auto-ethnographic experiences shaped the life history research, just as the life history work shaped my auto-ethnographic work.

The life history research I conducted involved learning from women who had reached their limits and/or stepped back from paid or unpaid caring roles in Ontario. As I will elaborate on in chapter 3, Ontario was a fitting site to situate this research as a setting contextualized by Canadian welfare state developments and demographic shifts. In our conversations together, research participants told stories about caring for others across the life-course – from babysitting, to caring for family members, raising kids, "clocking in" at group homes, day cares, or hospitals, and more. They also told stories about renegotiating care-related responsibilities and about rethinking gendered meanings and expectations. Their stories speak clearly to neoliberal privatization, market logics, and austerity policies that have put the onus on women, *in paid and unpaid care roles*, to shoulder the work and costs of care, and to figure out where they stand or what they think.

As a feminist sociologist, I link women's stories to material conditions in Ontario's care economy, as well as to dominant circulating narratives, assumptions, or expectations. Rebecca Schein (2014) writes that people's ways of understanding care provision are shaped through "individualist, market-based, privatized articulations" (173) that devalue the work of care and individualize responsibility for it. Elaborating on this, Braedley (2018) argues that our social and material circumstances may "limit our imagination and capacity to provide caring to frail older persons, as well as to welcome this care when we need it ... The inequitable underpinnings of capitalism deeply structure our experiences of care and caring (Luxton 1980, Luxton and Corman 2001), imbuing how we think about, plan for and organize care" (58).

In this project, it was important for me to examine how the social and material conditions of our lives deeply shape our vocabularies, imaginations, and the stories we tell. Stories represent, capture, and communicate dimensions of life (Doucet 2020). They tell us about how things are organized and hold invitations about how relationships and responsibilities are configured (Chivers 2013; Klostermann and Funk 2022).

As representations or "reflections," stories (including life stories) give meaningful form to experiences we have lived through, offering ways to "frame our understandings of raw, unorganized experience" (Garland-Thomson 2007, 122). Stories also "act" and "do things" (Frank 2010, 43), enabling us to create new meanings or ways of relating (Connell 2012; Frank 2010). We tell stories in the context of our lives and use stories to "make sense of – indeed, to act in – [our] lives" (Somers 1994, 618). Somers (1994) argues that "it is through narratives and narrativity that we come to know, understand, and make sense of the social world" and to "constitute our social identities" (606; see also Doucet 2018). Telling stories offers a way to reinforce or maintain our expressed subjectivities (Funk et al. 2019), as well as to reposition ourselves in relationships. Storytelling involves the "reiteration of classed, raced and gendered norms" (Byrne 2006, 1014), with dominant classist, racist, and sexist constructions existing in the imagination. Stories also have the potential to bring about new meanings and relationships, including more equitable or emancipatory ones (Basting 2020; Côté-Boucher et al. 2024).

Recognizing the power of stories, I weave approaches from the arts, humanities, and social sciences to attend to women's stories and to bring social imaginaries and relations of care to light in a different way. With my focus on intimate and institutionalized gender relations, and on the rhetorical work that women do in conversation to overcome perceived problems of persuasion (Klostermann 2019), I engage with and push forward research and thinking in feminist political economy.

Applying a feminist political economy lens helps me in attending to care as work and to divisions and relations between paid and unpaid work as shaped through social, political, and economic relations (Armstrong and Braedley 2013). The approach both recognizes the importance of care work in maintaining people and populations and recognizes that "there is a central friction, tension, or contradiction between social reproduction and capital accumulation" (Black 2020, 22; see also McWhinney and Braedley 2023). Such a lens supports researchers in tracing how gender, race, and class – as social relations, not only categories of difference – shape care work, and how the way care work is organized relies on and reinforces gender, race, and class inequities, as well as aged and abled norms (Armstrong and Braedley 2013; Bezanson and Luxton 2006). Feminist political economy supports with explicating oppressive social relations, such as those that privilege global capital development or profit-making, rely on separation or a hierarchy between men and women, and devalue the work of care (see Braedley 2013; Braedley and Luxton 2021; England and Dyck 2011; Vosko 2006). I am in good company with research in this tradition with my shared focus on examining women's work as it is organized, and with my goals of problematizing and transforming oppressive, capitalist, or patriarchal relations that perpetuate oppression along race, class, and gender lines.

I also note that research in feminist political economy primarily makes structural, macro arguments that put the focus on organizational or structural patterns and arrangements. Through comparative and context-specific inquiries, research tends to focus more on broader organizing conditions or social dynamics, with less attention paid to individuals' stories or strategies. One example of this tendency can be found in a recent article by Donna Baines and Pat Armstrong (2019), which claimed that not a single paid care worker that they interviewed as part of their research in over seventy long-term residential care facilities reported "wanting to care less or to avoid caring," with all workers reportedly wanting "to be able to care more" or undertake additional unpaid care beyond the work contract (7). While such an analysis captures dominant discourses and relations that relentlessly assign care work to women and strongly associate care with feminine and moral roles that are intrinsic to women, to me, it misses something about carers' agency or the various ways that people do innovate, renegotiate, or resist. It speaks to the need for research to "foreground the experiential" (Ferguson 2008, 48) and engage "with the specificities of agency, detail, and situation" (Code 2020, 39–40). It raises questions about the constructedness of people's stories, as well as the conditions under which some might be stripped of their "narrative range" (which is a phrase Litia Tuiburelevu uses, as cited by Lopesi 2021, 85).

In such scholarly accounts, differences in how people embody, make sense of, or resist care relations are less apparent. I don't mean this as a critique, as this work generatively explicates dominant social, political, or economic relations (such as those that relentlessly assign care work to women). But my goals here are different. In a project about transforming how we think, and with the research problems (and life problems) that I started out with, it was necessary for me to consider how women were actively interpreting and responding to the circumstances of their lives in the space of our conversations together and in relation to dominant gendered power relations and cultural frameworks. Alice Notley writes, "Staying alert to all the ways one is coerced into denying experience, sense and reason is a huge task" (1998b), and I think that was part of it. I wanted to interrogate my own assumptions, identify patterns and differences for women in different contexts, and look again at how stories get told and how we can tell new ones.

Every chapter is designed to produce clarity for feminist researchers, advocates, and students interested in gender and care work, as well as for those motivated to reflect on their own care experiences. I have a message that I think will be healing for others to read, including those who are currently in heavy caring roles as family carers or as paid workers in the helping professions. The book will be of particular interest to "former" carers or those who have committed to caring for others or to the making of a better world, only to experience a sense of disillusionment "at the limits."

I should say, my point with this book isn't to promote exiting care work. Nor is it to privilege workers' interests. I come to this work with an understanding of my own vulnerability and my own need for care as a woman with Marfan syndrome who underwent open-heart surgery at age thirty-one. It was in the second year of my PhD in sociology at Carleton that I was diagnosed with Marfan syndrome, and with an aortic aneurism, and told I needed an immediate abortion and open-heart surgery. I was also told that I would not be able to have kids. It was a whirlwind process that I've reflected on in the *Globe and Mail*, on the CBC, and in my one-woman performance show, *The Wounded Joker* (that is publicly available to view on YouTube). Forced into my body, I relied on the life-sustaining support of others. I spent five nights in the hospital following the eight-hour surgery, and another five nights when I experienced some complications. When I got home from the hospital the first time, I walked for two minutes the first day, and four minutes the next. Mine was a long and slow recovery, and I still live with the uncertainty of not knowing when or whether I'll need another surgery. These days, I flinch when I read headlines about the thousands of Canadians who have died on long wait-lists for surgeries, procedures, or diagnostic scans. When I see headlines of workers leaving the field or of long wait-lists for care, I know how hard it is for all involved. I know how much we need to get this right as a society, and how important it is to be able to rely on the life-sustaining care of others, with public investments to make that possible.

With that in mind, this book contributes to feminist scholarship and advocacy that challenges the ways that care work remains under-recognized, under-resourced, and unevenly distributed. I too push for ways of redistributing and revaluing care work. In speaking of progressive movements, Simon Black (2020) writes, "Typically, such projects involve demands for the state to socialize more of the costs of social reproduction and responsibilities for it, easing the burden on households and communities, especially the women in them" (23). When it comes to responding to problems of care, I am also inspired by Pat Armstrong's research and advocacy work. To give just one example, as the chair of the Women and Health Care Reform, a group funded by the Canadian federal government to identify and fill gaps in research on gender and care, Armstrong (who chaired the group for more than a decade beginning in the 1990s) worked with a small group of women from across Canada to raise questions and seek answers to four key questions: "Why is care a women's issue? What are the issues for women? For which women? What can we together do about it?" (Klostermann et al. 2022, 2). Her questions are ones that I take up here. Like her, I see working to investigate and transform care as a way to respond to issues of gender equity, as historically it's women – and primarily racialized, Indigenous, immigrant, and working-class women – shouldering the work *and costs* of care. My work contributes to these shared and ongoing efforts.

Without spoiling the plot, there are a few contributions I am most proud of. One strength of this book is in engaging with, and learning from, the stories of women in different age cohorts, class positions, and care contexts who told stories about negotiating responsibilities for care across the life-course. Looking at paid and unpaid care work, and at the stories of older and younger women, is a way to foster solidarity, putting my own life "in common with the lives of other people" (Silvia Federici as quoted by Vishmidt 2013). In future chapters, I read and present women's stories together – juxtaposing them, identifying patterns and contradictions, and revealing insights about the gendered power relations shaping and constraining their possibilities. There's no universal story here, and my attention to how context matters is another contribution. I take care to present deeply contextualized, *context-specific* accounts of women's lives, illustrating differences related to the nature of particular care relationships, work/organizational conditions, and the cultural pressures women faced at different social or historical junctures. Another contribution is in orienting to Ontario's care economy as a cultural context in which meanings and expectations around care are negotiated and remade, including through expressions of agency and resistance. I learn from women as political actors engaged in a politics of responsibility, considering how their insights adhere to and at times challenge dominant, hegemonic understandings of care. With a focus on the stories we tell, I attend to narrative silences, refrains, and tropes, revealing and rethinking the social and material conditions of their lives and the dominant cultural frameworks at play.

While care work is socially necessary, I argue that we need to rethink moral, feminine ideals that circulate and inform caring across the life-course, and that feminist researchers and advocates need new approaches to do so. My contributions to advancing methodological approaches to researching care are also worth flagging.

Advancing a Counter Politics of Care through Feminist Research

With its emergent methodology, this project involved experimenting with, enacting, and advancing what can be thought of as a "counter politics of care" approach. This included telling, eliciting, and learning from counter stories, as a way to reveal dimensions of social organization, identify dominant hegemonic understandings, and push for something more. I will elaborate throughout the book on the strategies I use, from embracing the power of stories; to reflecting on my own shared engagement with and implication in social relations of care and gender; telling fuller, more deeply contextualized stories; contextualizing and recontextualizing; and more.

My methodological approach combined in-depth life history interviews with auto-ethnographic memoir writing. Using auto-ethnographic writing as a sociological method offered me a way to situate myself in the research I was conducting, express sociological insights in an artistic form, and develop new and unexpected insights. I employed a sociological form of memoir writing in which one's "specific social context is very consciously brought into the mix" (Littler 2024, 2). With a feminist, equity-oriented approach (Winfield 2022a), I drew inspiration from feminist artist-researchers, including those who use memoir or other forms of creative expression (Carrier-Moisan 2020; Cvetkovich 2012; Hartman 2008; Keleta-Mae 2023; Littler 2024; Tamas 2011). In addition to writing in this way in chapter 1, I also weave in auto-ethnographic – or perhaps even confessional – insights in other chapters. My aim is to register complexities and convey the affective and intersubjective dimensions of my past work experiences and of my research encounters with participants.

With a confessional impulse to my work (Zucker 2023), I put myself on the line, writing about discomfort, shame, and confusion, while reflecting on my own "affective and ethical investments" (Cerwonka and Malkki 2008, 173). I include stories that don't always put myself in the best light, letting readers in on how I made my own missteps or projected onto others. I write about moments that felt cruel to be on the receiving end of, and moments where I felt cruel in how I responded to others. I share about times when participants rubbed me the wrong way, when they interjected to scold me, or when we jostled for moral position in conversation together. As a memoirist, this is an intentional way for me to investigate and make visible the complex terrain of women's relationships among ourselves, including by accounting for troubled intimacies and cruelty among women (see Taylor 2008).[1] I engage in "uncomfortable reflexivity" to be accountable to my own and others' struggles (Pillow 2003, 193; see also Visweswaran 1994).

When a mentor wrote in the margins of one part of the memoir that it sounded like I was raging in pain, I added a line to confirm that, yes, I was indeed raging in pain. With my goal of reflecting on how we can transform our interpretations, I reflect on my own shifting interpretations and my involvement in enacting and bringing about gendered relations and meanings. I slip in details about how I played a role in influencing participants' stories or in conditioning certain stories through the questions I asked or through laughter or other responses (Poletti 2011; Smith and Watson 1996). I also write about my own and others' agency, as we navigate, negotiate, and resist gendered power relations. I point to possibilities, reflecting on how my conversations with women shifted my own thinking.

The life history research I conducted centred on gaining insights into social life through exploring stories of how people "move through" life

---

1 My writing is in good company with the feminist memoirs that Judith Taylor (2008) analysed that use the first-person literary form to reckon "in house" or to problematize relations among women. Much like Taylor (2008), I orient to "women's sociality as imperative to the survival and development of feminism" (720) and "problematize women's social relations with one another within the frame of a feminist analysis" (710).

(Bryant and Schofield 2007). The aim was to reveal "the social" through an analysis of people's stories, linking those stories to the social relations and higher-level narratives shaping them. While "the life story is the 'story we tell about our life[,]' the life history is a collaborative venture, reviewing a wider range of evidence" (Goodson 1992, 6). The life history is the life story deeply contextualized within its social and historical context. And, while it is common for life history researchers to analyse people's "life stories" chronologically or with a focus on past practices in their everyday lives, I analysed not only the social practices participants told me about, but also their rhetorical practices in the interviews. This was important as one of my goals was to reflect on the cultural contexts in which meanings, expectations, and interpretations are negotiated and remade.

In total, I conducted twenty in-depth life history interviews with twelve Ontario-based participants, including eleven women and one trans, non-binary person, as part of a project centred on telling new stories about care and the limits of caring in Ontario. The interviews were conducted in the summer and fall of 2018, before the COVID-19 pandemic. I specified on the recruitment poster that I wanted to speak to "people with experiences reaching their limits and/or stepping back from a care responsibility or position in Ontario in some way (e.g., by sharing responsibility, finding other supports, resigning, or opting out)." While I was motivated to reflect on the "limits of care" or on "leaving care work," it seemed important to specify a *particular* care responsibility or position on the poster, rather than trying to recruit participants who had "exited care" once and for all or in general. It wasn't just that the concept of "leaving" didn't fully describe my topic, but that it didn't fully capture how people lived their lives, or how care demands can still be part of people's lives after leaving.

Taken together, the people who participated in my research had diverse care provision experiences (e.g., paid, unpaid, formal, informal, public, private, volunteer) in a range of contexts (e.g., homes, hospitals, day cares, residential group homes, live-in spiritual communities, shelters, long-term care facilities). Their stories weren't just about caring for their own children. They described inhabiting a range of care roles across their lives, including as family care providers (e.g., as children, siblings, spouses, partners, parents, grandparents), as informal care providers (e.g., babysitters, activists, volunteers, friends, doulas, care team members, camp counsellors), and as paid employees (e.g., direct care attendants, homeless shelter workers, support workers, therapists, social workers, nurses, teachers, day-care workers, live-in care workers, community service workers). Please see appendix 2 for a brief overview of participants' characteristics (age range, race/ethnicities, work/care histories, etc.).

Rather than focusing on care workers in a particular job (e.g., personal support workers) or particular care setting (e.g., group homes), my study design recognized forms and contexts of paid and unpaid care work as interconnected and interwoven (Doucet and Klostermann 2023). While sector-specific accounts of care in practice or carers at work are useful, I was motivated to respond to scholarly calls to attend to various kinds of caring work that women do throughout and across their lives in diverse paid and unpaid care contexts (Folbre et al. 2023). This was another contribution. It was also important given how paid and unpaid care work blends and melds across women's lives (Baines and Armstrong 2019; Duffy et al. 2015), for instance, with some women working double duty as paid care workers and unpaid carers in their households or communities (Doucet and Klostermann 2023).

As will become clear, there were differences in participants' social locations: rural and urban, single and partnered, parents and non-parents, younger and older, queer and straight, trans- and cisgendered, Indigenous and settlers, low- and high-income, and disabled and able-bodied. It's worth mentioning that I didn't exclusively recruit women, but no men signed up! Of note, I at times use the term "women" to refer to participants or to speak about how women are socialized into care. While I initially experimented with using gender-neutral terms such as "people" or "participants," I noticed that in trans participant Troy's own account, they themselves were making sense of the way they had been socialized into caring for others as an "oldest daughter" and as someone who was "A.F.A.B." (assigned female at birth). The term "woman," as it is used in this book, references those least likely to benefit from patriarchal forms of oppression (Eltahawy 2019). And again, my main focus is on revealing and rethinking gendered power relations through an analysis of participants' stories and strategies.

While I didn't set out to study age as I have in other research projects, it became important to do so as this study developed. Participants ranged from ages twenty-seven to seventy-eight at the time of the interviews (born between 1940 and 1991). While age groups are not homogenous, it became critical for me to analyse and call attention to patterns in the ways women in older and younger generational age cohorts[2] told

2 What constitutes an "age cohort" (e.g., such as young adulthood) relates "not only to chronological age, but also to developmental and experiential factors" (Silverman et al. 2020, 4). The term "cohort" refers to those born around the same time (and coming of age around the same time), and it is different from "generation," which refers to one's place in a family lineage (Katz 2017).

their stories. My point isn't that all women of a certain age have the same experiences or same ways of framing their lives. Far from it. But clear differences stood out to me, which led me to analyse how women who came of age in particular historical periods had different sorts of experiences and were exposed to different socio-cultural and conceptual narratives (see Mora 2006, 58–9). As we'll explore, one's age, phase in life, social background, or life-spanning experiences (such as of a recession, labour or economic conditions, or cultural and political currents) shapes and constrains one's practices, interpretations, and possibilities. As Pia Peltola and colleagues (2004) write, "As individuals pass from one life stage to another, their microlevel experiences and self-attitudes are influenced by the macro-level historical context" (124). It is also notable that the women who participated in my study were speaking from different vantage points; those in the so-called younger cohort (born after 1982) primarily reflected on more recent experiences of paid care work, while those in the older cohort (born before 1964) reflected on more recent experiences of late-life family caregiving. We can see in their stories how context matters, and I will highlight key patterns and differences in each findings chapter.

Most of the women I interviewed were white women who talked about their experiences in caring roles that seem to fit within the nurturance framework and with clear relational and emotional dimensions (Duffy 2005). The absence of racialized and immigrant respondents, or those in highly precarious, lower-paid positions, was a real limitation, and points to limits in my recruitment strategy and study design. When I first conceptualized the study, I conceived it as an auto-ethnographic project involving some research interviews in earlier phases. A mentor suggested that perhaps five interviews would be more than enough (given the nature of in-depth life history research that involves multiple long conversations with each participant). I was still taking baby steps to process my own personal trauma and wasn't dreaming that big at the time.

In saying that, the participant list raises questions both about who gets to exit care, and about whether some groups (such as migrant care workers) are harder to reach if engaged in other precarious employment following care. It's also notable that I recruited primarily through my own and others' contacts in rural and small-town settings where care facilities are known for being "white" and where further research is needed into the experiences of racialized workers in those contexts (Owusu 2019). Had I recruited through unions I may have been able to connect with paid workers in more diverse social locations.

In hindsight, I also suspect that some people didn't identify or self-select based on the recruitment criteria that specified "former care providers," as a few women whom I personally invited to participate indicated that they weren't sure they technically qualified since they had "opted out or stepped back" from some roles but were still engaged in others. Another possible barrier to recruitment was that on the poster I framed the study as a conceptual project to change the stories we tell about care. While tapping the shoulders of potential participants as storytellers and critical thinkers felt like a radical way to honour their insights, such an invitation may have implicitly addressed those in more privileged positions or with access to critical discourses. One participant mentioned having a panic attack before our session together as she wasn't sure what the dominant narratives around care were or whether she could challenge them. While I was quick to put her at ease, her comment speaks to the limitations of the recruitment strategy.

I also do question if, in some ways, interviewing white women with experience in care roles similar to the ones I had inhabited helped to create space for me to reckon "in house" or to experiment with more confessional, artistic modes of writing about the interviews that I conducted. A goal in my research was to push against some conventions in academic writing and to challenge some dominant ideals around women's selflessness, servitude, or discretion/secrecy in the context of care. I think it's worth considering whether using women's stories as memoir material or "fodder" for one's own healing and rethinking process would be appropriate for research with those in much more marginal, vulnerable, or precarious positions.

I will reflect more on how social relations of race, class, and gender variously shape and constrain people's options in the next chapter. You will also see in the findings that I work to produce a socially contextualized analysis of participants' stories. I make use of the in-depth life history research I conducted by telling "detailed and historicized" stories and "theorizing ... difference and particularity" (Steedman 1987, 16). In *Landscape for a Good Woman*, Carolyn Steedman (1987) refuses to look for universals experienced by all, but instead seeks to tell stories that are not central to dominant cultural accounts and that capture the particularities of people's lives. For example, she describes how her mother moved "a single bed, the television, [and] the calor-gas heater" (1) down to the kitchen when she was preparing to die, and how her grandmother had "six [looms] not because she was a good weaver, but because she was exploited" (31). Bringing context into view, she tells stories that can help us to "step into the landscape, and see ourselves" (24) and our lives more clearly. I strive to do the same.

With my goal of producing a well-situated and multilayered analysis, I didn't go through the interview transcripts to identify themes or pull quotes related to particular themes, but instead attended to how women told their stories, as well as to how the conditions of their lives shaped their practices and interpretations. I read and analysed each story in context, considering that person's formative life history and the social forces shaping their experiences. I also read and reread participants' stories in conversation with one another to identify patterns and differences (see also Ezawa 2016). Writing to think was central to my analytical approach.[3] In presenting my analysis, it was also a choice for me to present contrasting stories (e.g., of participants in different age cohorts, class positions, or paid and unpaid care roles) next to each other. You will notice that I juxtapose stories of care in different social and historical contexts as a way to show how context matters in shaping people's interpretations and options.

Outline of the Book

There is an arc to how this book is written, with my analysis of gendered care work unfolding as we go. In chapter 1, "Care Junkie Diaries," I presented a sociological memoir – written in a performative, literary mode – that focused on my own experiences as a care worker and an emerging care scholar. My auto-ethnographic account can be thought of as a "counter story." So, it's worth asking: What exactly is it running counter to? What is the dominant story of women and care? What are we up against? Chapter 3 – "What Stories Do We Tell about Care, and How Can We Tell New Ones?" – explores just that. Having introduced the problematics of the study and my feminist theoretical and methodological approach, I turn to introducing feminist scholarship that generatively situates women's care work experiences, paying special attention to race, class, gender, and morality. Reading about care's social organization sets the stage for the analysis that follows.

In chapter 4, "Reaching the Limits," I present a feminist rhetorical analysis of women's stories of reaching their limits in paid *and* unpaid care roles. With a focus on narrative silences and moralizing tropes, I

---

3 Inspired by Andrea Doucet and Natasha Mauthner's (2008) listening guide that can be used to examine questions of subjectivity or to attend to "knowing narrated subjects," I developed an expanded listening guide, which helped me to focus on, analyse, and *engage with* individual interview transcripts as (1) social texts or works of art; (2) life stories representing shifting configurations of practices over time; (3) relational encounters that we contributed to shaping in conversation; and (4) manifestations of "the social" that teach us about how their lives are organized. For more information on this process, and on the prompts that I used to engage with the data, see Klostermann (2021).

elaborate on the social functions certain tellings serve. One participant, Troy, commented that they could no longer "make water into wine anymore," and this captures a key finding, as participants narrated reaching their limits both as an embodied breaking point *and* as a moral achievement. My analysis in this chapter moves beyond mapping working conditions in uncaring organizations to call attention to women's shared implication in those relations and to dominant circulating narratives.

Chapter 5, "Loosening the Grip," engages with women's stories of leaving care work, with the goal of learning from women as political actors engaged in a politics of responsibility. I begin the chapter by looking at rhetorical conventions used for speaking about leaving, before shifting to considering how context matters (with some carers wiping their hands of certain responsibilities without thinking twice and others still digging their way out of it, years after). In attending to women's stories and strategies, I consider what they are up against and how things can be otherwise. I theorize care as a domain of struggle and rethink common-sense assumptions in feminist theoretical care scholarship.

In chapter 6, "Thinking 'Differently and More Deeply about Care Stories,'" I reflect on how hard it is to foster solidarity when there is no universal story about care work or womanhood, which then leads me to experiment with ways of telling more deeply contextualized stories of how conditions matter, with a focus on the nature of diverse care relationships, symbolic interpretations, and uneven work/organizational conditions. In comparing women's stories at different social and historical junctures, my analysis reveals shifting gendered power relations shaping how women enter into, inhabit, and make sense of caring roles.

In the conclusion, I summarize key contributions and their related implications. My final remarks stretch towards possibilities of how to foster solidarity among women positioned differently, as well as how to enact a counter politics of care and embrace possibilities for shifting or sharing responsibilities for care.

Chapter Three

What Stories Do We Tell about Care, and How Can We Tell New Ones?

Women Talking

From the fluorescent lights beaming to the plastic folding chairs set up in a circle, I have a strong image of what it would look like if the women in my study and I met in a community centre or maybe in the basement of a library to talk about caring for others. The theme of the event would be something like "What stories do we tell about care, and how can we tell new ones?" I'd have set out coffee and doughnuts and maybe something to go with hummus. I imagine myself coming on strong, with a provocative "we need to talk about the limits of care, let's lay it all out on the floor" pep talk to get things rolling. I would try *so* hard – rehearse long and hard – for a talk like that.

I'd likely lead off by sharing about my own experience as a care worker. "No one went under as I hard as I did," I'd joke. I'd want my story to register as unique and interesting, while secretly looking around the room and hoping that there'd be someone who saw herself in my story. On my feet and in front of the room, I'd speak back to the assumption that exiting care work is a "privilege" for "heartbreakers" walking off the job. The part that I'd most want to put on the record is how painful it had been for me to reach my limits and resign from the work. I'd share that I had committed to care as a vocation, had entered into the work to listen and learn from others and to build community, but that – over time and without the needed resources or supports to pull it off – I struggled to live out such a moral, feminine project. I'd emphasize that no longer being able to uphold the caring ideals that I had internalized felt like a crisis of self, something that I still struggled to make sense of or talk about. I'd express that I felt duped and betrayed, like I had been lured into care work with the promise of "moral becoming," only to have the rug pulled out from under me and be left with limited alternative scripts to affirm my worth or build a life around. To close, I'd suggest that we might learn from sharing and listening to women's counter stories, including the stories of women who could no longer hack it or who didn't want to do it anymore. "We should know the stories of our lives," I'd say. "So, um – can you – can you relate to my experience at all?" I'd ask, by way of inviting dialogue.

Drawing inspiration from Miriam Toews's *Women Talking* (2019) – an imagined response and work of fiction that sees women coming together to reckon with violence against women in their Mennonite community – I've thought a lot about how a meet-up between myself and the women who participated in my study might play out, with us variously positioning and distinguishing ourselves through our stories. There are conventions for speaking about care, and I suspect that we'd uphold them. Our conversation would likely sputter at first, like an old car trying to start.

If I had the ears of the women who participated in my study, I'd probably say something to try to bring us together or to point out some common ground between us. "I think maybe we have more in common than we usually recognize," I'd offer, looking around the room at older and younger women alike, who had worked in different helping roles. I'd be thrilled to tell them that no one I spoke with was a "type" of woman who said a specific "type" of thing. I'd mention that I interviewed activists, storytellers, and a woman who identified as a shit disturber. "Here's looking at you, Rhonda, you little shit disturber," I'd say. I'd also tell them about Vicki, a former AIDS activist in her early sixties, who had said, "I'm contradicting myself all the way through this." I'd suggest to them that Vicki curbed any reading of herself as a "type" of person who said a "type" of thing, and that others did too.

"Take Anne, for example," I'd offer. I'd tell them that when I asked Anne about her life-long commitment to care work and about whether she had "always had a sense of justice for sticking up to bullies," she nonchalantly said, "Oh, sometimes I was the bully. I used to be a bully. It was 50/50 at some points." I'd deliver Anne's response in a deadpan way, pausing for them to laugh. I'd mention that it seemed like Anne was challenging the idea that women are "born to care" (Stacey 2011) or have an affinity or identification with the role since girlhood. I'd suggest to them that some of their perspectives were quite different from carers in other studies who expressed only ever wanting to care more. I'd have to elaborate that there was more to it than any straightforward reading of them as living out normative, conventionally feminine positions or saying the type of thing that women say. "You each had unique and unexpected ways of putting it," I'd say.

I'd also share with them that I was thinking about how our stories change over time and how meeting with most of them more than once helped me to elicit contradictory stories and take "side angles." As I said to Carrie regarding setting up a second interview, "Maybe we'll have different parts of the story to explore. Maybe you'll remember something more, or we'll take a whole different side angle on it." I'd be sure to tell them how much my own story – or where I put the emphasis – changed through the process or even over the course of a single conversation. I'd mention that, when I first sat down with Anne, she shared that she used to work at a group home, to which I enthusiastically noted that I had as well and used to enjoy "jogging beside people on adaptive bike rides, coffee shop visits, making meals together, hanging out." We played our moral cards when we first sat down, but, as our conversation went on, Anne elaborated on how utterly exhausting caring had been, and I interjected to agree. "Yeah, yeah," I said. I shared that I too had burnt out, but that a story about jogging alongside others and enjoying it is the kind of thing you lead off with when you first meet someone. Anne burst out laughing, and it felt like we had found new ground together. "So, yeah, our stories change over time," I'd say.

I'd also want to tell them how much I valued the "work" we did in conversation together. "And I do see it as a form of work – actual work that tells us about how our lives are organized and what we're up against," I'd say. I'd tell them that, when I first turned on the audio recorder for my interview with Nora, a paid care worker around my age who was born in the 1980s and was in her thirties at the time of speaking, I excitedly announced in a sportscaster voice, "All right. Okay. We're rolling. It's July 24th and we are chatting about care." From there, with the recorder on, Nora teased that now "we had to perform and say all the right things," but that I could "edit the awkwardness out." We let on we were making a future something, and I even joked to Nora that it was like "a bad reality TV episode." But our conversation involved "work" that can teach us about the circumstances of our lives, and the gendered power relations at play.

"There was pleasure in the research process," I'd announce to the room. Rasing my coffee, I'd tell them how I laughed throughout my conversation with Nora, and how I laughed when I first turned on the audio recorder with Carrie, and she leaned in, licked her lips, and jokingly announced, "I hereby give Janna permission to record this interview." She said it in an overly formal, theatrical way, poking fun at the process. "Okay, uh, thanks," I had responded, blushing. "And *we are* off," I added. Our conversations were sites of creativity, meaning-making, and even fun. They were political spaces that we entered into as political actors engaged in a broader politics of responsibility. "The work we did together in conversation matters," I'd say. "And I think we'd make one hell of a reality TV show if we had the chance."

Maple cream doughnut in hand, I'd want them to know that no two participants had the same experience. "It's been really powerful to talk to people who have had different relationships or trajectories or where it's maybe not as straightforward as what I had in mind," I'd say. I'd admit that I had a particular narrative arc in mind when thinking about women and care. "Mine was a pretty romantic one: service corps, care work, went downhill, burned out, stepped away. So, a pretty clean narrative in terms of writing a movie," I'd say. "You have the climax." I'd have to explain that some women's accounts bulged at the seams, with stories of fits and blasts, entrances and exits, and overlapping care responsibilities along the way. "Different scripts, plot points, narrative arcs," I'd say. "A real shitshow to analyse, quite frankly." I'd want them to know that I'd been working hard to challenge some of own assumptions, that their stories had been helping the cause.

But as I picture it, we'd find ourselves pitted against each other right quick. We'd hardly have time to finish our coffee! I picture the elite, happy-go-lucky good girls with empowered stories to tell about caring on one side of the room, with me and the other care junkies or dupes, emphasizing our resentment and bitterness, on the other. I picture one of the good gals, purring, "I *loved* caring for others, came through well and whole and in one piece, and can't understand why *they're* so bitter." On the other side of the room, I picture one of my care cronies sarcastically quipping, "Fun, fun, fun," before joking about going over the care cliff and hardly being able to recognize herself when she was done with the work. "Must be friggin' nice to have pulled it off," she'd say. I imagine that we'd all stand back, imposing on one another the "cultural meanings [our] historical moment required" (Garland-Thomson 2017, 39). More than a passive, innocent spectator holding a clipboard and watching it go to crap from afar, I'd likely be taking the bait, rolling my eyes at some of the sentimental accounts, wondering how on earth to put my stories in common with the stories of others.

With stories touching stories, the wide range of ways in which women in my study framed their lives and positioned themselves in relation to "care" tells us something. The tropes we reached for were revealing. And although the scene above was an imagined one, it speaks to some patterns and contradictions we'll explore in the coming chapters. In a disruptive, counter-story-telling research project, not everyone framed themselves as resisting inequitable care relations or challenging moral, gendered imperatives for women to care against all odds. The women

I interviewed didn't say a "type" of thing, but there were some common refrains, tropes, or narrative silences. Even in a study about the "limits of care," some were hesitant to go there, or seemed bent on trying to present themselves as ideal caring women. Attending to these differences – to how we set ourselves apart – became part of my task. As a feminist sociologist, I worked to put our lives in common, to attend to patterns, differences, and contradictions, and to contextualize our stories in relation to the material conditions and conceptual narratives shaping them. Silvia Federici (2012) writes, "We need to put our lives in common with the lives of other people to have movements that are solid and do not rise up and then dissipate" (70). Contextualizing and recontextualizing women's stories was central to my work, with a range of feminist scholarship offering the theoretical tools needed to direct my attention.

In what follows, I introduce some of that scholarship as it situates women's stories of paid and unpaid care work. We'll look head-on at divisions and relations of labour (e.g., that assign and value care work along race, class, and gender lines) and at ideals around femininity, morality, and whiteness. To close, I'll present some research on care conditions in Ontario, where I conducted my research.

Situating Stories of Women and Care

A range of feminist scholarship highlights how girls and women are funnelled into caring roles, how care relationships are organized and institutionalized, and how care is valued or what it means. The social organization of care "refers to the location of this work, the conditions of those who provide it, and the value the work is accorded (Glenn 2010)" (Black 2020, 24). It is an important concept in feminist care scholarship, as it recognizes how one's situated social, material, and historical location matters, while directing attention to organizing conditions and valuations.

With a focus on oppressed groups, feminist sociologists of care work consider how girls and women are coerced and conditioned into providing care, making visible how race, gender, class, and citizenship status operate as central organizing forces in valuing and assigning care work tasks and responsibilities (Dodson and Luttrell 2011; Duffy 2011; Glenn 2010). Not only is care devalued as feminized labour (Baines and Daly 2015), "low-income and minority groups tend to bear an unequal share of the burden and costs of care" and tend to have higher needs for care, for instance, with higher rates of chronic illnesses or disabilities (Levitsky 2014, 8).

In her book *Forced to Care*, Evelyn Nakano Glenn (2010) writes that "the social organization of care has been rooted in diverse forms of coercion that have induced women to assume responsibility for caring for family members and that have tracked poor, racial minority, and immigrant women into positions entailing caring for others" (5). Glenn pays particular attention to how race operates, elaborating on how whiteness, which is linked to power and moral superiority, is central to capitalist accumulation and to the exclusions and harms experienced by women and people of colour.

With global divisions of labour, care work is assigned to women, or immigrant, racialized, and working-class women in particular (Chun and Cranford 2018). As researchers observe, women are funnelled into paid care work roles in organizations typecasting for care positions, tugging at their heartstrings, or playing up the emotional rewards (Palmer and Eveline 2012). Feminized sectors where women "choose" to work are often lower paid (Armstrong 2007), with such choices not "a matter of unconstrained will," but rather "heavily conditioned by structural social arrangements that impose limits on what women can do" (Wajcman 2000, 188). Given how care is naturalized as the domain of women, there is little recognition of the skills involved (see Armstrong 2013). There also isn't much recognition of how women enter into that work with limited alternative labour market options (Dodson and Luttrell 2011). Scholars also raise questions about the extent to which family carers' unpaid work is entirely voluntary (Armstrong and Klostermann 2023; Funk 2015) or the extent to which volunteering is a choice (Overgaard 2019). Womanhood is associated with family-making, with women sometimes viewed as becoming or perhaps only counting as women when they are acting as wives or moms.

While broader social relations socialize men and women differently in relation to care work, there are differences in the nature of care work or what it entails. Mignon Duffy (2005) distinguishes between caring roles that fit within the "nurturance framework" and have clear relational and emotional dimensions, and "reproductive labour," which includes lesser-valued, low-wage, low-status dirty work. When it comes to how care varies by context, it's also notable that the ways of inhabiting caring roles described by women in my study were quite different from the figures of "differential surrogates" or "professional others," which were subject positions produced through caregiver recruitment and training programs in Taiwan and Japan (Lan 2016).

To give another example of how context matters, in Canadian nursing homes, which are typically large-scale, hospital-like institutions, care aides support with task-based, bodily care work, in contrast to care aides in Sweden, who support with all aspects of daily living, including laundry, meals, and medications (Armstrong et al. 2009; see also Storm and Lowndes 2021). Notably, public spending for elder care is three times lower in Canada than in Sweden (Storm and Lowndes 2021), with care aides in Canada supporting up to twenty residents per shift compared to nine residents per shift in Sweden (Daly and Szebehely 2012). Indeed, the political and economic conditions shaping what we mean by care matter.

Speaking to this, Albert Banerjee and colleagues (2012) found differences in levels of violence experienced by long-term care staff in Canada and Scandinavian countries. They write, "When the proportion of careworkers experiencing violence on a daily basis is compared, Canadian frontline careworkers report six times more physical violence (43.0% compared to 6.6%), four times more verbal violence (35.5% compared to 7.4%), and twenty-three times more unwanted sexual attention than their Scandinavian counterparts (14.3% compared to 0.6%)" (394). In their study, they used the concept of "structural violence" to point to organizational and systemic relations shaping how care relationships play out. It isn't that older adults in Canada are more aggressive, but that different conditions shape how care plays out. As Pat Armstrong and other scholars remind us, "the conditions of work are the conditions of care" (Armstrong et al. 2020, 7). This also applies to "working" conditions for family carers, with some care scholars even using the word "workers" to refer to unpaid family caregivers and to remind us that their working conditions and protections matter too (see Cranford 2020; Streeter 2023).

Just as the work of care varies by context, so too do gendered expectations and meanings around care, femininity, and morality.

A range of research reveals how dominant assumptions frame care as an intrinsic feminine capacity or activity, as well as the assumed expectation of girls and women (Braedley 2015). Through normative upbringings and admonitions related to care that frame it as a feminine activity (Braedley 2015), society has worked to produce girls and women who willingly assume their gender roles and undertake gender-assigned duties and obligations for care, including in their households and in paid work (Glenn 2010, 43). As Susan Braedley (2013) writes, "Exposed to these messages and the admonition that *good women* care for others and especially for their families, girls grow up amenable to uncompensated or low-paid care work as an opportunity to attain feminine moral worth" (60). Relatedly, Laura Funk et al. (2019) call attention to "dominant conceptions of gender roles, whereby caring activities are connected with caring identities which provide self worth and a sense of self" (6). Caring historically has strong links to the normative feminine position, which has traditionally involved being passive or at least not assertive, while accommodating, supporting, or nurturing others (Gilligan 1982; Ringrose and Renold 2010; Skeggs 2001). Good girls ought to care.

In Western cultural contexts, caring is associated with moral goodness, responsibility, or relationality, while not caring is associated with being selfish or privileged. Such formulations have roots in Judaeo-Christian perspectives claiming that "the obligation to care for others is in conflict with selfish desires" (Hollway 2006, 113). A moral dimension enters into the equation when one has a sense of good/ bad, right/wrong, or what one "ought" to do, as well as a sense of how they think others in their community would perceive or judge their actions (Doucet 2006, 186). Morality is embodied, constructed, sustained, and ordered in relationships between persons (Eicher-Catt 2005). That which is "moral" is contextually specific and socially/culturally mediated – brought about in context and in relation to larger public moral visions or evaluative frames (Doucet 2006; Kelly 1998; Levitsky 2014; Walker 1997).

One place where care is moralized is in feminist care scholarship that underscores our shared need for care and the relational nature of our existence. In feminist care ethic literature, care is understood as socially necessary and central to a just society, with society understood as having a moral obligation to provide care. Feminist care ethicists forward relational perspectives of care that challenge notions of liberal, autonomous "individuals," recognize vulnerabilities and dependencies as central to the human condition, and acknowledge care as central to social and political life (see Gilligan 1982; Kittay 1999; Tronto 1993). They take seriously that people deserve to have their care needs met, and that we need to ensure the democratic provision of care for those who need it (Tronto 1993, 2013). Moving beyond an ethic of justice, research in the tradition argues that care relations offer a basis from which to constitute an ethic for political philosophy for democratic life. Recent developments in ethics of care literature further underscore our relational nature – challenging normative understandings of care, while elaborating on how care relationships are shaped through oppressive histories of colonialism and capitalism (FitzGerald 2020; Robinson 2011). Studies also show how care is shaped transnationally, including in the contemporary contexts of neoliberalism, global politics, and human security (Mahon and Robinson 2011; Onuki 2011; Robinson 2011).

In regards to societal moral expectations, girls learn early that caring for others has moral significance, and they work to position themselves in relation to that assumption. Experiences of caring for others are interwoven with "people's identities as moral beings," which are actively "constructed, confirmed and reconstructed" (Finch and Mason 1992, 170). What it means to be "caring" is wrapped up with ideas about what makes a "good" woman, mother, daughter, person, or care worker in particular social and historical contexts. There is a personal and public dimension to cultivating morality, as we internalize expectations in caring roles (Ruddick 1995) and negotiate our sense of ourselves as moral beings in relation to ourselves, others, and social expectations (Doucet 2006). We also see this dominant assumption at play when "women who abandon family values and selfishly pursue new lifestyles of their own" face criticism (Ezawa and Fujiwara 2005, 46).

That said, there are discrepancies in the ways care as a moral practice is valued or understood in public discourse (Funk et al. 2024). Public discourse at times valorizes or idealizes care by framing carers as heroes or saints. At other times, caring at the individual level is associated with less desirable traits (e.g., martyring, controlling, over-mothering). For instance, in some media portrayals, care workers are framed as abusive, all-powerful, morally compromised individuals, with limited attention to institutional contexts that devalue people who need care and commodify care practices (Lanoix 2005).

Public moral visions or imaginaries valorize, idolize, and elevate some figures, while criminalizing or stigmatizing others as "threats" to social values (Cohen 1980, 9). We see this with the Madonna/whore divide, which distinguishes between good, morally pure women, and those who are bad, promiscuous, or selfish. There are also distinctions between "good" and "bad" mothers. As Molly Ladd-Taylor (2004) observes, in a study of the cultural politics of mother blame and worship, "You can't have a 'good mother' – at least the way the dominant culture defines her, as selfless, nurturing, and true – without a bad mother to compare her to" (7).

Elaborating on this, Alicia Ostriker (1986) writes, "Good motherhood ... is selfless, cheerful, and deodorized. It does not include resentment, anger, violence, alienation, disappointment, grief, fear, exhaustion – or erotic pleasure. It is ahistorical and apolitical" (179). Ostriker gets at the rigid social expectations at play, with expectations around selflessness, decorum, and modesty. A carer is one who looks after the needs of another – eases their burdens, tends to them. There are limits on her voice and around the visibility she can bring to her experiences. There's an implied separation between the independent, autonomous, powerful carer and the dependent, vulnerable recipient (see FitzGerald 2020). There's also an assumption that carers have their own needs met and have the capacity to meet others' needs.

In situating women's experiences, feminist scholars also direct attention to racialized divisions and labour market disadvantages related to race or citizenship. The care sector is stratified along lines of gender, race, class, and immigration status, with hierarchies between women (Cranford 2020). We can see this in Canadian nursing homes, where most workers are women, but racialized immigrant workers are over-represented in more precarious, low-paying, and lower-status positions (Owusu 2023; Syed 2020). With less anchoring in Canada's labour market than other groups have (Block and Galabuzi 2011), racialized immigrant workers are subject to deskilling and have fewer opportunities for employment mobility, with policies that don't recognize foreign credentials or that require workers to stay in the same positions on temporary work permits or remain working until old age (Lightman 2019; Lightman and Akbary 2023; Syed 2020).

Transnational care circuits unevenly distribute resources globally and over-rely on migrant women care workers (Gottfried and Chun 2018; Mahon and Robinson 2011). Undocumented workers in particular are positioned as more easily exploitable through social policies and are more likely to work in the informal care economy where they are seen by some employers as "cheaper" or more likely to put up with being mistreated (Thomas 2023).

In her study of undocumented Caribbean care workers in the United States and Canada, Carieta Thomas (2023) highlights how racist and stereotypical depictions of Caribbean women powerfully shape the choices they make. Caught up in a "respectability" politics, some try to do things the "right" way, which can also lead to them policing other members of their ethnocultural group or wanting others to follow the rules. So, while some women can easily be positioned as "ideal carers," others continually need to prove their respectability. For instance, racialized workers in nursing homes face additional pressures to constitute themselves as "proper" workers or prove they can do a good job (Storm and Lowndes 2021). They are often less likely to raise problematic issues around racist or unwelcome treatment (Storm and Lowndes 2021) and less likely to be able to set limits or say no (see Klostermann and Funk 2024). We can also see how racial hierarchies are negotiated and resisted in practice – for instance, in the case of Filipina live-in caregivers agentively negotiating cultural stereotypes others have of them (Pratt 2000; Gardiner Barber 2000).

I explored in chapter 1 how, as a white woman with Canadian citizenship, my "respectability" and "goodness" weren't in question, or at least not to the same extent as others I worked with. In her book *Poetics of Wrongness*, Rachel Zucker (2023) questions whether her whiteness makes it possible for her to be bad on the page or write about a "fall from grace" in a vulnerable way that might elicit sympathy. She introduces the insights of Shane McCrae, who writes that "the assumption behind it [confessional writing] is that grace is the default position. For writers of colour, it is not assumed that grace is our default position – we are always tainted by the sin of being oppressed" (McCrae as cited by Zucker 2023, 64). As Zucker writes, "If confessionalism is built on the premise that only white people can fall from grace and that people of colour are already 'fallen,' then the confessional designation is a white supremacist construction because it relies upon the notion that only white people occupy a state of grace from which to fall" (64). Her remarks offer an important lens for interpreting some of the counter stories I present in this book. They speak to the importance of interrogating and analysing conceptions or constructions of whiteness that underpin care arrangements and cultural ideals of care.

It's also important to consider how femininity as a pure, moral project usually references or is seen as the project of a "white, Western, middle-class woman" (Beverley 2011, 152; see also Yelin 2016, 185), with care imagined as the domain of white women. It is *white* femininity that has historically been a position of moral superiority, with white women expected to domineer over racially marked others (Schaffer 2019, 91). Speaking to this, Evelyn Nakano Glenn (2010) attends in her book to "racialized servitude," with women of colour coerced to care, and others commanding their services. She gives the historical example of African American communities' own efforts to "reform" Black women or provide vocational courses in domestic training as a way to work against racist stereotypes of Black women as sexually promiscuous.

Caring for others can be a privilege for some who have the resources needed to pull it off, a burden for others who are conscripted or coerced into care, and a missed opportunity for those who are prevented from caring all together. As Emily Abel (2000) writes, "poor women, especially women of colour, historically have had to struggle to care for intimates" (8–9) and have been prevented from caring. Black women have been denied the roles of mothers or the privilege of caring (Zucker 2023). In Canada, colonial and ableist legacies and realities have prevented Indigenous families from caring for their children or communities, while disabled people have also been refused the right to care or prevented from having children.

When looking at stepping back, we also need to consider who is stepping in, as well as how people are left responding to care gaps that hit some communities harder than others. We can see how this played out with the pandemic, as, when some opted out of formal work, a racialized and gendered workforce of immigrant and migrant workers were called on to work in hazardous conditions, and with limited access to worker protections (see Das Gupta 2020).

Social relations of race, class, gender, and citizenship profoundly shape how care plays out, and the stories presented in this book need to be considered in light of these wider oppressive histories and realities.

Care Conditions in Ontario

Given there's no universal, ahistorical, apolitical story of care, it's important for me to say more about care conditions in Ontario, Canada, as they are organized through specific social policies. As we'll further consider, what "care" looks like, how one comes to provide it, and whether people can access it is a matter of design.

As is the case across Canada, the restructuring and devaluation of Ontario's care sector has given rise to deepening and intensifying issues. There have been stories of inadequate care levels and unmet care needs, facility closures and service suspensions, and long waitlists for nursing homes, day cares, and other forms of care (Armstrong and Braedley 2023; Wells 2020). Insufficient investments in publicly provided health or social care services are noticeable in tensions and scandals and in violence, accident, and injury rates (Armstrong et al. 2019; Banerjee et al. 2012; Lloyd et al. 2014). Paid care workers and unpaid carers alike have been exposed to physical and psychological hazards (Braedley et al. 2018; Grey et al. 2018), with real costs and consequences for those who provide and rely on care. There are problems in long-term care, childcare, disability services, and other care-related sectors.

Yet these problems aren't new. Across Ontario, the care economy has been acutely strained for decades. Long-standing public underinvestments in care work and privatization measures have put the onus on individuals to meet their own care needs. It was in a 2002 article, *over twenty years ago*, that Jane Aronson (2002) gave the example of a home care case manager advising a client to recruit a neighbour to help with her evening eye drops (409). The onus of responsibility for having one's own care needs met was assigned to that individual, with a built-in policy assumption that care should/can be provided by families or that people have a daughter to do it.

With the eye drops as one example, provincial governments have forwarded neoliberal agendas over the last few decades in Ontario. These agendas can be linked to the Harris Conservative government cutbacks in the 1990s and are evident in the ways that subsequent Ontario provincial governments have continued to privatize care and limit the scope and responsibility of the welfare state (Daly 2015; Joseph and Skinner 2012). Constrained public welfare spending, along with the ongoing restructuring of care services, have framed care provision as a private responsibility (e.g., of individuals, households, communities, or the voluntary sector) and have led to people relying on the private market or on for-profit or private forms of care (Armstrong and Armstrong 2019; Daly 2015; Skinner et al. 2016).

It's this shifting of responsibility from the state to individuals – with the state withdrawing responsibility for care or downloading care onto individuals – that is of particular concern to feminist care researchers (Black 2020). In the chapters that follow, we see the over-reliance on women's unpaid contributions in their stories of supporting friends or family members in their households and communities (Klostermann and Funk 2022; Streeter 2023) and in their stories of doing unpaid work at work, such as by working through breaks, coming in early, or staying late at organizations without clear boundaries (see Klostermann and Funk 2024).

It's notable that most women who participated in my study had experiences providing paid *and* unpaid care across their lives, which again speaks to how women are often "hit twice" with cuts in the public sector and with more work being sent to households or families (Braedley 2015). With clear links to inadequate public sector investments, paid staff *and* unpaid/family care providers have been required to "pick up the slack" or compensate for systemic issues by performing unpaid work or working long hours for low wages (Armstrong 2023). This is again about austerity agendas that lead to inadequate or diminished public services, which create gaps in care to be filled by women's unpaid or underpaid labour. The over-reliance on unpaid work in particular is a form of privatization, as it involves a shift from public or state-provided support to the private provision of support (see Armstrong and Armstrong 2019).

With a focus on women's care-negotiation strategies, and on the stories that they tell, we will look in future chapters at paid and unpaid work across contexts and across the life-course. We'll orient to Ontario's care economy as a cultural context in which meanings and expectations around care are negotiated and remade, including through expressions of agency and resistance.

Chapter Four

Reaching the Limits: Inequitable Care Conditions and the Moral, Feminine Impossible

This chapter presents a feminist analysis of women's stories of reaching their limits. I explore how the way we talk about these experiences can either keep gendered power dynamics in place or flip them on their heads. We all tell ourselves stories about our lives, shaping our identities and making sense of our experiences. These stories, often laden with cultural and social expectations, can either reinforce dominant narratives or challenge them. My focus in this chapter is on analysing women's stories of hitting their limits, and analysing the silences in their stories, to reveal deeper social and moral implications.

But this chapter also does a bit more than that on a personal level. Midway through conducting my research with other women, my therapist suggested that I had reactivated the trauma that I had experienced as a care worker, inflaming old wounds. After such a traumatizing experience, it was hard to set down the story or snap out of it. I felt sick thinking of how much I had been exploited by the organizations I had worked for, and of how society had put me in that position, devaluing my life to that extent. Sure, that was part of it, but I also felt sick thinking back to how I had crossed ethical lines – power-struggling with the people I supported and coming to see *them* as part of my problem. I couldn't get over how turned in on myself, and on the experience, I had been. As an embodied researcher (Baines et al. 2024; Ellingson 2017), I was in the midst of my own grieving process, wrestling with feelings of sadness, anger, guilt, shame, and confusion.

This was vulnerable research (see Winfield 2022b), and my questions about care's limits were ones I was profoundly motivated to explore. With real stakes, and with a commitment to rethinking and reflecting on my own interpretations, I wanted to learn from how others made sense of reaching their limits. I wondered: Had they too been turned in on themselves and others, struggling to see outside the experience?

Had they crossed lines, confronted a different side of themselves? What about disgust, resentment, or regret? Had they found ways to hold things in a lighter way or to have more compassion for their historical selves? Could we learn from one another, get somewhere together in conversation? As a memoirist and former carer, I was hungry to learn from research participants on a personal, radically selfish level. I was also curious, as a sociologist, how their stories might help with disrupting dominant, hegemonic understandings of care and with filling out empirical understandings of care's social organization.

When I first started exploring these questions and trying to make sense of women's experiences, a range of feminist care scholarship helped me to consider issues around burn-out and around the psychological health and safety hazards faced by paid care staff and unpaid care providers (Braedley et al. 2018; Grey et al. 2018). This research considers how such hazards are brought about through organizational, political, and economic relations, which can lead to care providers experiencing physical and psychological harms (Banerjee et al. 2012; Brassolotto et al. 2020; Grigorovich and Kontos 2019). Of particular note, Susan Braedley and colleagues (2018) attend to how "working conditions [in long-term residential care] are determined at the policy level as well as by owners and managers," and with "jurisdictionally specific funding and regulatory regimes" (92). "We're told, 'Suck it up. It's your job'" (91) was how one care worker in their study put it. The authors argue that work and occupational hazards (such as work overload, discrimination, and rates of accident, violence, and injury) *are structural problems*. They also make the important point that structural conditions and processes need to change. In this chapter, I build on that work by learning not just from workers in a particular sector, but from care providers across a range of paid and unpaid care contexts. Further, beyond a focus on people's everyday work experiences, I look closely at the constructedness of their stories.

In the analysis that follows, I attend to women's stories about reaching their limits or confronting hazardous conditions, with a focus on the rhetorical conventions they used as they overcame perceived problems of persuasion in telling their stories. All of this is a way to reveal "the social." I'll first start by looking at narrative silences around the topic of limits, or how women's stories were shaped by silences (Blix et al. 2021), before then tracing moralizing tropes in women's stories. As I'll illustrate, the work that women did as they framed their lives can be understood as a form of "moral, feminine work," as it involved negotiating their moral, gendered sense of selves or self-expectations and positioning themselves as respectable in relation to others. I will also consider how women's stories speak to intimate, closer-in attachments or entanglements in care relationships that they themselves were part of and implicated in.

In considering below how women's stories serve to establish their respectability, I draw inspiration from research on feminine practices of distinction. In her research on sex workers in Ponta Negra, Brazil, Marie-Eve Carrier-Moisan (2015) found that women tried to establish their respectability or embody their roles in respectable fashions through feminine practices of distinction. Such embodied and discursive practices weren't just about managing stigma or rejecting particular labels or their negative connotations; they were ways of actively producing oneself as respectable. Following Carrier-Moisan (2015), we can see in the narrative silences and in the moral, gendered tropes that I analyse below how women were actively positioning themselves as (moral, feminine) subjects through claims of respectability.

In regards to the moral dimensions at play, it's notable that while participants didn't always reference "morality" directly, they did express moral dimensions in making comparisons to others, in talking about right, wrong, good, and bad (or what one should do), and in depicting moral emotions such as guilt, shame, anxiety, or embarrassment (Santoro 2018). We can also see in women's stories how morality is socially mediated and actively negotiated (see Doucet 2006; Santoro 2019; Zigon 2013), as they put effort into constituting their moral lives or responding to moral concerns, such as by "experimenting" in relation to their social personhood or relationships (Mattingly 2014).

"A moral breakdown," Jarrett Zigon (2013) writes, "is an experience of self-reflection during which persons must ethically work on themselves in order to transform their moral subjectivity, even if ever so slightly, so that they can return to the everydayness of their life trajectory" (211). I appreciate Zigon's perspective – that a moral breakdown involves self-reflection and working on oneself – and I pay attention in this chapter to how people do such work in conversation. In focusing on moral dimensions at play, I challenge the dominant, hegemonic idea that care relationships grant moral status to carers who are coming from more privileged positions, claiming power over the people they support. While it is indeed the case that care relationships can be oppressive to those who need care, we also see in women's stories how moralized understandings of care can contribute to holding carers captive – setting the stage for their own depletion and harm, while negatively impacting all involved.

Narrative Silences: Did It Rattle You as Well or Do You Remember ...?

When I shared my recruitment poster with my doctoral committee member Janet Siltanen, she commented that it was like a blunt instrument – a powerful way for me to direct and frame my research as a counter-story-telling project. I couldn't have agreed more! On the poster, I framed it as a project that aimed to tell new stories about care and the limits of caring in Ontario. I didn't play coy or pretend it was an open-ended study to learn from people's experiences or to explore "what care meant to them," but I instead directed my focus. Razor-sharp. I mentioned on the poster that I wanted to learn from people who had "experiences reaching their limits and/or stepping back from a care responsibility or position." I also let it slip that I had skin in the game, noting on the poster that I was a former care worker. I was proud of that little poster. I even included an image of a woman "walking away" on it. In the face of scholarly research that aims to retain nurses and other paid care workers (Ben-Ahmed and Bourgeault 2023; Devi et al. 2021), I liked that there was a bit of a "flinch factor" with my topic. I felt like a shit disturber sending the poster around. It also meant something each and every time someone responded to express their interest in participating. Hearing from other women brightened my day.

But – *well, how should I put this?* – in a study about the limits of care, I learned quickly that it was hard for some to, well, talk about the limits. There were narrative silences, as this was not something some wanted on the record. My conversation with Gracie provides an example of what I mean. She spoke in a bubbly and upbeat way and introduced herself as a "pretty normal fifty-five-year-old woman" (born in the 1960s) when I first turned on the recorder. Gracie was a former family caregiver and current administrative assistant. "Nobody would have been able to care the way that I did," Gracie said. As she told story after story about *excelling* at caring for others, I wondered why she had signed up to take part in my research. "Always a caregiver, just became a part of me," Gracie said. She narrated a lifetime of caring for others out of the goodness of her heart, from raising her two kids, to running a home day care when they were young, and providing direct daily care both for her mom (following a heart attack) and for her husband (following a stroke). Gracie said that she didn't have a choice and had to care and be selfless, but that she always felt "satisfied" and "content" and "rewarded" for what she was doing. "Soothing souls" made her happy.

"Fabulous, it was just fabulous," Gracie said to me, in speaking of the care she used to provide. She *reminisced* about soothing souls and framed caring for others as an act of love, central to who she was. In speaking of operating that home day care when her kids were young, Gracie said it had been a "fabulous job" and noted that "if you have more kids than you have hands, it doesn't really matter how many more you have." It sounded to me like a cover-up. I couldn't help but notice that she brushed over the skilled work involved. She didn't say a whiff about her family's financial situation or about the lack of access to publicly funded child-care options in Ontario at that time. She didn't mention that it had been cheaper for her to open the day care than to pay for childcare for her two kids. It seemed to me like she was mystifying care, keeping women from knowing the stories of our lives. "Just fabulous," Gracie had said. And, again, I wondered why she had signed up.

Finally, after eighty minutes in conversation together, Gracie mentioned that her mother's major heart attack and recovery process had rattled her son to the core, and I sheepishly interjected to ask, "Did it rattle you as well or do you remember ...?" I squeaked out the question. I felt like a shit disturber for asking it, as though I was messing with her self-image or posing a threat to the story that she was telling about herself. Her story was one about caring accomplishments she was proud of and that her family still praises her for. In response to my question, Gracie confessed that she was at her "wit's end" from sleeping with the baby monitor on and "living one big adrenaline rush all day and all night." But, from there, as if not wanting to go one bit further, she underscored that she came through "well and whole and in one piece." It seemed to be her way of saying "nothing to see here" or "no need to explore that topic." *Hmm* ...

I had a similar experience struggling to broach my research topic in conversation with Judy, a woman born in the 1940s, who was in her seventies when we met. Judy welcomed me into her rural home, served tea, and affectionately teased me for ringing her neighbour's doorbell after I had gone to the wrong house. I also teased Judy after she mentioned being raised in a Pentecostal home and not being able to wear make-up growing up. "I see a little lipstick now," I said, smiling. Similar to Gracie, Judy was proud of the care she had provided across her life. The word "blessed" was a refrain in her account, as she narrated a history of finding enjoyment in caring for others, starting with supporting her frail mom and baby sister growing up, to raising her kids and providing late-life care. Even in speaking of supporting her husband, who had cancer, and her dad, who had dementia, *at the same time*, Judy emphasized just how grateful and blessed she had been. She even said how blessed she was to have a care aide sit with her husband for three hours a day so that she could visit her father in long-term care during that time. "*Aww*, busy year and a half then," I commented to Judy. I let out a deep exhale as I said it. I said it like "whew" or "well, shit, eh?" or "*gosh*, no wonder you signed up to participate in a project about limits!" But even after I tried to create space for Judy to talk about any challenges, she doubled down by emphasizing how rewarding caring for others had been. "So I had to be strong and be the caregiver," she said. "But I accepted that challenge, because I just found it so rewarding."

Eventually, after ninety minutes in conversation with Judy, I shuffled my notes, cleared my throat, and asked, "One of the things I put on the poster was about reaching your limits. Can you relate to that in any way?" I passively attributed my interest in the limits of care to my recruitment poster, as though I hadn't made the poster myself and as though I didn't want to be the type of woman to try to elicit an uncaring counter story by my own volition. I couldn't even spit out the question myself or ask it in a way that might seem like it was one I wanted to ask: "On the poster I sent, it says ..." By way of responding, Judy mentioned that the *only* time she reached her limits was when she wasn't allowed to visit her husband after his surgery, as the nurse had said, "no more visits tonight." I mean, *my goodness!* My question about limits was purposefully vague in that I hoped to open up or invite alternative meanings (beyond a narrow focus on "burn-out"), but I didn't expect such a question to be used to reinforce a narrative about how she had excelled as a moral, feminine caring subject and had just wanted to care more. *Hmm again ...*

To give just one more example, I also struggled to broach the topic in conversation with Sheila, a family caregiver born in the 1950s, who was in her late sixties when we spoke. Sheila and I met in a coffee shop on a hot summer day. She waltzed in wearing a beautiful all-white linen outfit, as I sat a bit sweaty in an Eddie Bauer athletic dress with bike shorts underneath. To her credit, or perhaps I should say our credit, it took me only thirty-five minutes to raise the topic of limits with her, so that was sort of a win. But only just *sort of*. Although I had been able to edge in with a question about the limits of care, Sheila's response to that question was likewise just a blip in a bigger conversation about the exemplary care she had provided to her mother. In speaking of reaching her limits, Sheila said, "We were coping with a lot at that time. It was just starting to be a bit overwhelming." She didn't say that she herself was overwhelmed, but that *they* (meaning she and her husband) were coping and *it* was just *starting* to be a bit overwhelming. She spoke in the "we" and without any regrets. It was a "starting to be a bit" and a collective "we." So, *hmm!* Sheila had let it slip that it had been all-encompassing, 24/7 care, and that she had slept with a baby monitor on, so I had to wonder, why was she radiating gratitude?

Eventually, after working up the nerve, I asked Sheila, "I ended up feeling quite resentful when I reached my limits, and I'm wondering if there was – if you felt that?" My hands shook as I asked the question. It felt like my way of asking whether she could imagine what it was like for me or appreciate how I felt or how I had been set up. The question had an ethical demand. With a demure fluttering of her eyelashes, or as if the thought had not occurred to her, Sheila responded, quizzically, "[You're asking] if I had felt resentful? No. No." She repeated the word "no" twice and in a delicate and soft way with a pause in between each one, as if taking time to carefully consider it. "I realize I made sacrifices," Sheila said, "but I wouldn't have done it differently." At the time, Sheila's response stung. To me, it seemed like she was bent on telling an empowering personal story, maintaining the pretence of the caring institution, or upholding a culture of secrecy, as I was still licking my wounds and processing my own traumatic experience as a care worker.

In my conversations with Gracie, Judy, and Sheila, reaching one's limits seemed like a touchy or taboo topic. It was framed as a little, wee blip in life histories of caring well for people they loved. It seemed to go against the grain of the stories they were telling, as they only very briefly elaborated on that part of the story after being prompted by me. There were silences there. And as Bodil Blix and colleagues (2021) write, rather than trying to get people to break their silences, it can be important to honour and try to understand them. The task is to be "wakeful to the silences in and between people's stories, to the silences in our own lives, and to the functions the silences may serve in both our own and others' lives" (592).

While I noticed silences in some interviews, in others I hardly had time to turn on the audio recorder before the person I was speaking to interjected with a story about reaching their limits. With a sense of narrative urgency (Luttrell 2000), some *rushed* to put that part on the record, as they told stories about depletion, harm, or their own missteps.

Gina, a disabled woman and family carer in her sixties (born in the 1950s), was quick to mention power-struggling with her mother and how much she had resented the requests that came her way. Some days she had wanted to kill her. "I was a grown woman; I didn't need my mother telling me what to do," Gina expressed, fuming. Hers was a story of being pit against the person she supported. In a way that speaks to the severity of her situation, Gina also told me that she wanted her kids to "pull the plug" on her, rather than seeing them suffer the way she did as a care provider. "Never. Not in a million years," she said. "I know what [they'd] have to go through to keep me just breathing; it's too much to ask of any person." To me, Gina's comments spoke to how her own imagination for care had been diminished through the work given how inequitably organized it had been. Others also talked about becoming turned in on the situation or struggling to see outside of it. They put the tacky or taboo parts on record.

Nora, a paid care worker who was around my age (born in the 1980s and in her thirties at the time of speaking), shared about reaching her limits and finding it hard to be around some of the people she supported. Clearing space for her to tell a counter story, I asked, "Can you remember what irritated you about [the people you supported] at the time?" Nora responded, saying, "Just, like, people's needs." She said it with a bit of a giggle. She also stated, "I started kind of tuning out more or, like, I'd get more short-tempered. I was power-struggling more with them or feeling really resentful and angry." She said that she just tried to "get through the shift," but "started feeling angry towards them and more just, like, just dislike towards them and resentful and stuff like that." While Nora spoke in an authorial, first-person voice when describing caring for others, she at times hedged, trailed off, or addressed a generic "you" in speaking of reaching her limits: "almost," "sort of," and "kind of," like when "you" would "just [be] kind of shitty," when "you" are impatient or stressed. These were harder stories to tell, ones she seemed to need a bit of distance from. This also seemed to be a way for her to position herself as part of a group of like-minded people, as someone who wasn't alone in her reactions.

So, some seemed to align with dominant, hegemonic understandings of care, while others seemed to resist them, or at least that's what I thought at first. On the surface, the conversations I had with some women, in which I found it hard to broach the topic (Gracie, Judy, Sheila, Marilyn), seem to clash or contrast with the stories of other women (Carrie, Nora, Troy, Gina, Rhonda). Yet, as we will explore further, some of their stories served similar social functions, helping them to reinforce respectable moral, feminine positions or to do "moral, feminine work." Having looked at narrative silences, we'll now look at moralizing tropes.

Moralizing Tropes: Reaching One's Limits as an Embodied Breaking Point and Moral, Feminine Achievement

Women variously framed reaching their limits as an embodied breaking point, a moral, feminine achievement or outcome of having sacrificed, and a source of guilt or shame. Troy, a former paid care worker, said, "I don't know how to make wine out of water anymore," while Gina recalled caring for her mother, saying, "I guess none of them [siblings] could do that. Because I did. They were not willing to give up their life for her. None of them." With powerful statements to really land the sentiment, they both expressed reaching their limits as a breaking point, *as well as* a moral achievement or outcome of having done the impossible as direct carers. They claimed power through tales of disempowering experiences, positioning themselves as respectable, moral subjects through their stories. There was a contradiction there. As we'll explore, calling attention to one's body giving out or to one's good intentions or guilty feelings can be a way of establishing one's respectability by signalling that one values care or is aware of moral imperatives to care. In such stories, the dissonance and discomfort expressed suggests a "recognition of dominant expectations about care and gender that were not being followed and therefore required explanation" (Aronson 1998, 124).

The Body Says "No"

"A body can stop functioning," Sara Ahmed (2020) writes. "A body can announce a complaint." Several women in this study emphasized that they wanted to continue caring, but *their bodies* just said "no." Taken together, they called attention to life-altering health experiences or embodied signs: exhaustion, depression, anxiety, weight loss, high blood pressure, dizziness, spinal injuries, sciatica, back pain, chronic pain, and chronic headaches. As some told it, their ingrained moral expectations of what makes a good woman or caregiver were so intense that it was only when their bodies physically started coming apart – when they felt they had reached their physical limits – that they felt that they had sufficient moral reasoning or justification to step back from care or go against the grain of what they thought made a good person. Stories about the body saying no seemed to offer them a way to position themselves as respectable moral subjects, while also releasing themselves from moral expectations to continue providing care in that context.

Anne described an intensely physical experience and extreme situation that led her to make the difficult decision to drop her disabled son off at developmental services when she and her husband could no longer care for him at home. She didn't mention her year of birth, but I would guess that she was in her early fifties and perhaps born in the mid-1960s. It stood out to me that Anne's story was a political advocacy tool (Panitch 2012). She emphasized that there had been a "major problem in the system itself" and that it had been a "three-year wait-list to get an assessment" for her son. With such inadequate social policies in Ontario, her son "aged out" of social services support at age eighteen and was no longer eligible for publicly funded support, although he still required around-the-clock care. Anne elaborated that she feared for her son's life. She also mentioned that she and her husband were sleep-deprived, stressed, and burnt out from providing around the clock care and going up the echelons to advocate. Like others, Anne emphasized that she had wanted to continue caring but couldn't physically do so. She said, "I had blood pressure – 220 over 115, and, you know, normal blood pressure is like 120 over 80 or 90. So, I was up into the area where you can get a stroke, brain aneurism, heart attack. Quite frankly, I was petrified of my own health."

What caught my attention in Anne's story was her reflection that the burden of saying no or setting limits on the care that she could provide wasn't something she considered, or something that felt possible, until her own body gave out. As she told it, she had wanted to continue caring but couldn't at her physical limits. And even if that's just how she told the story, I think her story tells us something about dominant conditions getting in the way of women being able to share responsibility or set limits on the care they can provide.

Carrie, who was introduced in chapter 2 and in her thirties when we spoke, also described an intensely physical experience and extreme situation that led to her reaching her limits (in her case, as both a mother and paid care worker). "So *that* was the breaking point," Carrie said. She recalled a "life or death" turning point in which she underwent a "mental break" and experienced her entire life grinding to a halt after years of caring for people who "didn't have their shit together." Cracking jokes to cope, Carrie said, "I would finish work, pick [the kids] up, and I'd be driving home and just crying ... from exhaustion. I'm a weirdo. I get really tired, I cry. My eyes just leak. And I get pale. Eyeball vampire!" In addition to disassociating and passing out at Walmart, she remembered passing out and waking up on the floor at home with her dogs licking her face. "I'd just come down to get a drink, you know, and wake up. *Frig!*" Her story was one of having had her body say no, at an absolute, extreme breaking point, which also seemed to give her the permission she needed to renegotiate expectations to care that she had previously upheld. Her bodily complaints were measures of seriousness and indicators of stress in a care sector that can be disabling for care workers, who are often women working "double duty" with care responsibilities on and off the clock.

"It rattled me terribly; it did. That was the very first time in my life that I ever went to see a professional counsellor myself," Gracie said. Born in the 1960s, Gracie talked about care experiences across her life, including a more recent experience providing direct daily care after her mother's heart attack. While she was hesitant to tell this part of the story about her limits, and it seemed to go against the grain of where she was putting the emphasis, she did elaborate on how the experience took a toll. Gracie stated that she was at her "wit's end, very overwhelmed, very sad." She was completely and utterly exhausted. "And the exhaustion," she emphasized, "the exhaustion ..." She also said, "My hands would shake without me telling them to." While Gracie fit the memory into a narrative of how she was a caring person, and felt the experience had strengthened her, hers was also a story about reaching an embodied breaking point at the limits of care. Similar to others, hitting her physical limits seemed to give her the permission she needed to seek out some help and ask for more support from others.

In the stories told by Anne, Carrie, and Gracie, emphasizing an absolute breaking point in an extreme situation seemed to be a way to position oneself as a respectable, moral subject who wanted to continue caring, and would have cared against all odds, but didn't have a choice. As they told it, it wasn't that they didn't want to care; it was that they reached a physical limit or the body said no. Similar to reports of "female disposability" observed in feminist studies of the workplace (Wright 2001), the stories of women in different age cohorts and different care contexts underline how inequitably organized care can be in paid and unpaid care realms. Their stories reveal normative moral ideals (or assumptions around what one "ought" to do) in relation to which these women were tasked with positioning themselves. To me, this idea – that it is only when one's body literally shuts down or one has a near-death health crisis that one has sufficient moral reasoning or an argument that is strong enough to go against their socialization of what makes a moral person – shows how much is getting in the way of women being able to resist hazardous conditions or tell stories to challenge them head-on.

People That Care the Most

A second related trope that was used by paid and unpaid carers in different age cohorts was to frame "reaching one's limits" as a moral, feminine accomplishment or outcome of having invested or sacrificed. We saw this in the stories above, about turning water into wine or giving up one's life. Another clear example of this is found in a comment by Nora. "The people that care the most end up getting the most fucked over," Nora said, laughing. She framed burning out as evidence of how well-meaning and caring she had been. Like Nora, paid and unpaid carers in different age cohorts employed this convention, framing reaching their limits as an accomplishment, while emphasizing both how much they had cared and how well-meaning they had been. Employing this trope also seemed to offer a way to distinguish oneself as a respectable moral subject who had been committed to feminized care work but was moving in a different direction.

Troy, who was in their thirties when we spoke, remembered feeling like they didn't have the energy or emotions, or couldn't even take care of themselves, when they resigned from their work at a homeless service centre. They had only just resigned a few weeks before we spoke. Like others, they described *their body* as the one who was calling the shots. As Troy said, "My body has been telling me in bizarre ways: 'No, you don't have energy for this; go take care of yourself.'" Troy also recalled their doctor telling them they were having a "chronic stress reaction," and that they needed to fill out a WSIB (Workplace Safety and Insurance Board) incident report. Their body said no. Yet, what was most striking to me was how Troy framed reaching their limits as an accomplishment of sorts. Conjuring up images of the idealized, youthful, relational care they used to provide, Troy reminisced about going above and beyond with trips to parks, playgrounds, and the beach with the service users they supported. They mentioned how they used to "get told how young and bouncy and fun" they were, how they had been "kind of like Mary Poppins," and how they had been "attached" and like "family" to the people they supported.

Speaking with a hint of bravado, and in a way that I related to, Troy shared about the disembodied, self-sacrificial care they used to provide, when they would "forget to eat and forget to go to the bathroom" and would just be "there and totally present with someone." Not being able to care *any longer* was linked to a history of caring well. "My approach and my caregiving roles are different from a lot of co-workers [who are hard and jaded]," Troy said. "But I think it also explains why I'm kind of burnt out now." Telling it this way seemed to offer a way to position themselves as a moral, caring subject who honourably went in "with [their] whole self all the time" but could no longer do so. It's sure hard to simply tell a story about reaching one's limits without needing to qualify one's self-worth or distinguish oneself from others, isn't it?

Sheila, a former government director, who had waltzed in in that linen outfit and was in her sixties when we spoke, also framed caring as a moral, feminine accomplishment in speaking of reaching her limits and placing her mother into a private retirement home near her house. Sheila underscored how caring and well-meaning she had been, asking, "Did I take too good care of her?" She also recalled that even her family doctor had said, "Your mother wouldn't have lived this long if it hadn't been for you." While Troy talked about playgrounds and park hang-outs as a paid care worker, Sheila recounted magical summer holidays at the cottage, kids sitting on her mom's lap, card parties, costumes, and skits. I laughed when Sheila mentioned how her mom trick-or-treated at her front door shortly after moving into the granny suite in Sheila's home. "You couldn't tell it was her in the Halloween costume, until she brought her cane around," Sheila said, laughing. She also expressed, "We mostly just say, 'If Granny were here, she would be doing ...,' you know, depending on what the situation is." It struck me that she infused her story with anecdotes about what a great relationship she had with her mother. Similar to Troy, Sheila drew a clear line between her history of caring well and her experience struggling and needing to set limits by placing her mother in residential care.

Troy and Sheila described care in different contexts. Troy clocked in at work. Sheila supported her mother both at home and in a private retirement residence. Yet, in the stories they told, they both linked reaching their limits to histories of caring well and to how well-meaning they had been. Others framed it this way too. I know I did. At times it was as though our experiences of exhaustion or overwhelm were something to be proud of, evidence of what good, caring subjects we were. And, even if that's just how we come to tell these stories, it sure tells us something about gendered power relations getting in the way of us being able to protect our own health and well-being or challenge the hazards of the work. Such stories speak to material conditions of care and to the culturally sanctioned exploitation and subordination of women. They need to be challenged and rethought. I must ask: Why is it so hard to tell a story about inequitable conditions of care without clarifying what kind of a well-meaning, caring person one is? Why can't we tell a story about hazards or limits full stop?

Guilt on Top of That

A third moralizing trope was in women's expressions of guilt – of having felt guilty, of still feeling guilty, of being hit with a sense of guilt just talking about reaching one's limits. Guilt can be thought of as a moral emotion that is backed by cultural norms and feeling rules (Donath 2015). It has long had an association with caring or with good mothering in particular; as Aminatta Forna (1999) puts it, speaking of motherhood, "the guiltier the better" (76). Relatedly, Orna Donath (2015) argues that accounts of regretting motherhood "indicate the intensity of the social and cultural mechanisms that institutionalize the path toward good womanhood and good mothering" (345).

With few exceptions, and with "caring about" strongly equated with "caring for" (Davidson 2015), women in this study talked about feeling guilty about reaching their limits and no longer being able to care for others. Similar to the stories we looked at previously, women's guilt-ridden stories of reaching their limits have clear moral dimensions, conveying the tremendous social pressure they felt in relation to imperatives to care for others. In speaking of feeling guilty, Julie, a paid care worker born in the 1990s and in her late twenties when we spoke, shared, "I don't think [my co-workers] felt guilty because they would just never do [the pampered bath routine or little extras] and they never really would notice the difference." Her story seemed to offer a way to distinguish herself from others. We will also see below how expressions of guilt can help women create space to move in different directions or release themselves from expectations to provide care. Such stories seemed to be a way of saying, "I can't do it, but I'm aware of moral expectations enough to feel guilty."

In speaking of reaching her limits, Gina, a disabled woman in her sixties, expressed feeling like she had done something wrong that necessitated feeling guilty or ashamed. "Fun, fun, fun" was a cynical and sarcastic refrain in her story. She narrated lived experiences of disadvantage, including tumultuous family relationships, violence in a previous marriage, and health issues such as long-term physical disability, chronic pain, and mental health issues. She said that she was forced to shut down her home day care to become a full-time caregiver for her mother, and she was still bitter about how her family had left her stranded, providing full-time, 24/7 care to her mother for eight months straight. She was one of several participants who talked about feeling guilty about reaching her limits and no longer being able to care for others anymore. "Guilt on top of that" was how she put it. She said she felt "totally guilty" and "extremely guilty," as she reported no longer being able to care for others, including her grandchild. Gina said, "I feel horrible saying that. Just saying that makes me cringe, because I'm supposed to want that. It's my job to want that. But I don't want to do much as a grandmother. I just, I don't want to do it. It's 24/7 caregiving again, and I don't want to do it. It sounds horrible, doesn't it? The more I say it, I feel horrible."

At the time of speaking, Gina was still wrestling with guilt and still working to reorient to herself and to self-expectations she had previously held. "Does that sound bad?" was a question she asked a few times. Continually calling attention to guilt seemed to be a way for Gina to express a sense of herself as a moral person, who had wanted to continue caring for others but no longer could. "I feel horrible even talking about it," she said. She attached moral value to caring as something she was supposed to want, and as something she saw as part of her job as a grandmother, but created space for herself to move in a different way, limiting the direct care she could provide.

Guilt was also a thread in Nora's account of reaching her limits and resigning from paid care work at a residential group home, where she had supported adults with developmental disabilities. Nora, who was in her thirties at the time we spoke, had worked at a group home for several years in the 2010s when she was in her late twenties, and had resigned a few years before our conversation. Like Troy, she was a feminist thinker in her own right; she had an analysis of ageism, ableism, and of the ways feminized care work is devalued. Throughout her account and in different ways, Nora emphasized how guilty she felt about reaching her limits and no longer being able to care for others. As she said, "I didn't want to leave the work, because I was so immersed in it ... I still felt so guilty and so tied to it ... I didn't really know who I was without it." She attached moral significance to caring as something to feel guilty about not doing. She underscored her guilty feelings and heartfelt desire to care more, with her story providing moral justification or a way to (re)constitute herself as a moral subject – someone who cares enough to feel guilty about not caring.

Gina and Nora spoke about care in different contexts and had different ways of putting it. Gina referenced expectations for grandmothers. Nora referenced her desire to live out disability politics by sharing power and learning from people with developmental disabilities. Yet, they both did moral work in conversation, as they expressed feeling guilty about reaching their limits and no longer being able to care for others. With stories that served similar social functions, they both attached moral significance to caring, as something that was integral to them and that they felt guilty about not doing. The intensity of their accounts suggests they had internalized social expectations to care in the contexts they were in.

Rethinking Moral Captivity, Even If That's Just How the Story Gets Told

My analysis speaks to how one's moral sense of self can be put on the line, and implicated, even when invited to speak about "reaching one's limits." There were clear narrative silences and moralizing tropes in the stories above. When asked about reaching their limits, women in this study variously dodged the question or took care to reinforce their sense of self-worth or express their moral, feminine commitments, as if that was what was in question. Their stories reveal a profoundly moral terrain and raise questions about how to keep women in caring roles safe or create space for talking about hazardous care conditions or personal limits, without feeling like one's sense of self is on the line. It's worth asking why we feel the need to qualify our self-worth through stories of exploitative conditions, and how we could change that.

I have to say, when I first started analysing women's stories of reaching their limits, I was tempted to draw a bit of distance from them by signalling to the reader – an elite imagined reader, perhaps – that I was well aware of the ways *they* had upheld dominant, hegemonic narratives of care, or the ways *they* had over-internalized responsibility, pushing it until *their* bodies said no with *their* good intentions or *their* guilty feelings. Yet, with my "counter politics of care" approach, I have tried to open myself up to learning from others through this research. I also have to say that I resonate with the stories women told and have employed similar rhetorical conventions in my own stories.

In one of my three conversations with Troy, they asked me, "So, *uh*, do you think you'll go back to caregiving? Or do you feel like you have to step away from it for, like, a really long time?" Their question caught me off guard. "Yeah, um, it's, um, yeah," I said, sputtering. "I guess lately I've been – or, like, for a while felt like I needed to, like, get away full stop or like I could hardly even face it or even with my – I, like, felt …" I stuttered in my response at first, but eventually used all three of the moralizing tropes that I identified in the stories of other women. I mentioned that I still value care, that I still felt a lot of guilt about not caring, and that I couldn't physically sustain it, as I had been blackout drunk a couple nights a week as a care worker. *Check, check, check.* At the time, I didn't realize that such lines – about my body giving out, about my good intentions, and about still feeling guilty – were tropes that other women in this study also relied on. I too positioned myself in relation to moral "oughts," re-establishing my moral sense of self in the stories I trotted out. My response to Troy illustrates how I had internalized expectations to care for others and how I was still wrapped up in moral, feminine ideals five years after resigning.

What I want to underscore here is how moralized understandings of care can contribute to holding carers captive – setting the stage for our own depletion and harm, while negatively impacting all involved.

Judy's account of distinguishing herself from others offers an example of what I mean. "There are people who put their loved ones in long-term care homes and don't see them or see them maybe once a week, but I couldn't do that to my dad," Judy said. She distinguished herself from others who she felt didn't provide adequate care. To give another example, she remembered confronting a PSW (personal support worker) who was employed at her dad's nursing home, saying in a stern voice, "That is deplorable." Smugly (and in a way that made me cringe), Judy commented that the "little PSW ... softened after a while." Through what Yen Le Espiritu (2001) refers to as "ethnic boundary practices," Judy reinforced divisions between herself and others to "reconstruct a sense of value and self-worth in the context of racial and ethnic subordination" (Kim 2018, 1048). As Judy said, "She [the PSW] – maybe in her culture and her ethnic background – she wasn't taught that [how to provide proper care], you know, maybe she didn't know. Maybe that's her mannerism."

With a distancing account, Judy in some ways got a leg up over racialized and ethnic paid workers. As Andrew Sayer (2005) writes, within a moral economy, "social groups often distinguish themselves from others in terms of moral differences, claiming for themselves certain virtues which others are held to lack" (953). Judy indeed distinguished herself from others – legitimating her belonging to a caring life project, while making uncaring, racialized subjects into the problem and using them as objects from which to draw her "own moral value, purity, and distance" (Wood 2018, 636; see also Dosekun 2020). I can see how problematic that is. Indeed, the way that care is moralized, set apart, or made into a white project of distinction needs to be interrogated from an antiracist perspective. Furthermore, what this chapter illustrates is how the ways in which these moral ideals circulate and inform care contribute to making *carers themselves vulnerable*. It isn't just that they embody and enact oppressive histories and realities (see Williams 2010), but that they themselves are made vulnerable through those histories and realities. If no one else can do it or there's no other moral way to live, and you're locked right in there, that might be the "special" place to be, but it's a recipe for disaster too.

To give another example, Nora talked about struggling to step back after reaching her limits. She mentioned that she had a savings account, had housing options, and could have technically left, but *still* struggled to move on. Nora said, "I was in such bad shape, like I couldn't have physically or emotionally even been there anymore. My body literally, you know, gave out on me." She also mentioned that her "mental health wasn't good, but, even then, it was still so hard to leave." With care as something that was central to who she was, part of what seemed to keep Nora captive, and what can contribute to inadequate care (in situations where people stay to the point of power-struggling), was the way her moral sense of self and self-worth had been wrapped up in the work. It's worth asking: What does it say when a person is at their limits, has the material resources needed to leave – housing, employment options, or savings – but is too attached to the idea of themselves as a particular kind of person to simply walk away?

Troy also spoke to the moral imperatives to care that had led them to stay past the point of reaching their limits, and to experience a real rupture when they could no longer sustain the work. Troy framed resigning as a way to ensure they didn't become the "worker no one wants," like their "hard and jaded" co-workers who would "just half-ass" it or "do the bare minimum" or "set boundaries" or "delegate" without really helping anyone. Like Nora, what most seemed at stake in Troy's story was who they were as a person. At the limits of care, *that* was the part that seemed most weighted:

> It just kind of happened so fast. And I think I just wasn't present enough to even figure out what was happening in the moment ... I went into my boss's office, and I just said, "Please don't hate me." And she's like, "What?" And I'm like, "I can't hear you," and I just kept saying, "Please don't hate me, please don't hate me, please don't hate me." And she just shut the door and was like, "What's going on." And I handed her the [WSIB] papers and she's like, "Oh, okay, so you're not working anymore. How are you?"

With "please don't hate me" as a refrain, Troy spoke to how caring, as a moral and political commitment, had been wrapped up with their sense of self-worth. At stake in their story was their sense of belonging. Reaching their limits and no longer being able to care had been an intimate, profoundly threatening experience. And as we will contemplate in future chapters, such a story speaks to the need for ensuring care providers have options and avenues for meaning, self-worth, and belonging, outside of dead-end paths or traps that can take so much from them.

In saying that, and as Troy's story highlights, it wasn't that care providers were completely stuck or held captive. Some of the tropes we looked at were tropes that travel. As we've explored, stories about our bodies saying no or about our own good intentions or guilty feelings seem to offer us ways to move in different directions or to release ourselves from the weight of moral expectations. For instance, whether in speaking of a body that can't hack it or expressing a sense of guilt, women often expressed regret that they no longer had the capacity to care, and in turn weren't someone who should be counted on or put in that position again. "I wish I could, but I can't." These were tropes that travel. In the context of women's lives, such stories helped them to move in a different direction. If trapped or guilty were the two options, it seems that, rather than staying trapped for life, the stories women told were ways to reposition themselves. When Gina asked, "I mean, do you have to almost die before you start taking care of yourself?" she seemed to speak back to the idea that carers don't have needs or that care should be a death sentence. It was a question to challenge exploitative conditions, a way to get somewhere.

Final Thoughts

Care conditions matter. In women's stories, there were clear links to neoliberal privatization, market logics, and austerity policies that have put the onus on women, *in paid and unpaid care roles*, to shoulder the work of care, and the work of trying to meet their own needs or find ways to frame their experiences. The conditions of our lives deeply shape our vocabularies, imaginations, and the stories we tell. Without a doubt, there are real social and organizational factors that contribute to psychological health and safety hazards and lead some carers to reach their physical and psychological limits (Braedley et al. 2018). These embodied, material conditions, which are about diminished public-sector supports for care, need to be addressed to support and ensure the safety of both those who provide care and those who need care. We can see the dangers, for care relationships and people's well-being, when carers have limited options to step back or share responsibility. We can also see how hard it is for women to *even talk about* their personal limits, or about hazardous conditions that reinforce their subordination, which is evident in their narrative silences and in the tropes that they use to qualify their moral self-worth.

Women's rhetorical practices reveal a profoundly moral/cultural terrain in which one's sense of self is on the line. No one told a straightforward story of uncaring working conditions or organizational and structural dynamics without also elaborating on intimate, closer-in attachments or entanglements in care relationships of which they were a part of and implicated in. There wasn't one account of simply being exploited or violated that didn't also include some work to justify one's life choices, make something of oneself, or signal moral commitments that were important to them. These stories speak to the stronghold of normative ideals around morality, care, and femininity that "formalise and entrench a set of unviable subject positions" (Ringrose and Renold 2010, 583). And, even if that is just how we came to tell our stories, that too says something about what's getting in the way of creating equitable conditions or having frank conversations about hazardous conditions or shared struggles among women.

My analysis suggests the "ethic to care," at the individual level, can hold women in exploitative relationships. Women's stories speak to how "moral injunctions, not to act unfairly toward others, and *not to turn away* from someone in need" (Gilligan 1982, 20, emphasis added) can be quite constraining when pushed to the limit in wider conditions of social neglect or without options for individuals to share responsibility. We saw this with Anne, Carrie, Nora, Troy, and others. With all hands on deck to retain care workers or "care for the caregiver" to ensure she can keep going, women's stories underscore how important it is to rethink gendered power relations to ensure women can leave and can talk about their needs. Further, I think the claim that carers are somehow benefitting from morally superior positions in relation to vulnerable others misses something important about the ways some carers can be held morally captive, with real costs and consequences for all involved. Women's counter stories challenge that dominant assumption, showing how that moral bind can be part of what makes it hard to keep themselves and others safe (see Clifford Simplican 2015).

Stories of carers pushed past the brink, with their own bodies saying no – whether through shaking hands or dangerously high blood pressure – underscore the importance of ensuring that care providers, in paid and unpaid roles, and in a range of contexts, have options to exit when needed. Likewise, stories from women hemming and hawing or struggling to talk about the limits of care point to the need for expanding social imaginaries to ensure women's safety and well-being. Having explored women's stories of reaching their limits, we'll now turn to examining stories of stepping back from caring roles and relationships. We'll further consider moral, feminine meanings and relations that can make care work hard to leave. We'll also learn from how women, as political actors, develop strategies to resist and renegotiate.

Chapter Five

Loosening the Grip: Reimagined "Care Ethics" and the Politics of Responsibility

The historical story of domestic services describes jobs that women leave when they can. One scholar of nineteenth century domestic service [Sutherland 1981, 61] observed: "In most cases only people in desperate financial straits, those who considered service a brief interlude to better things, or those who could not find employment elsewhere became servants."

– Duffy (2011, 33)

The phrase "women leave when they can" suggests they stayed only as long as they had to in domestic service jobs, with clear links to their social and material circumstances. It's also notable that the political and economic conditions that restrict women's employment opportunities – leading them into care work in the first place – shape and constrain their options for leaving (Duffy 2011; see also Dodson and Luttrell 2011). When recruitment into paid work happens in the context of choosing between working and starving (Irving 2017), those conditions also impact one's ability to leave. Indeed, it's important to account for the material or structural relations shaping and constraining people's choices.

That said, the idea that it is a privilege to exit, or that it is privileged women who exit, is something that I challenge head-on in this chapter, with a focus on women's stories of leaving, stepping back from, or otherwise renegotiating responsibilities for care. The idea that it's a privilege to exit is also something that I heard again and again when I first started conducting research on the topic of exiting. We saw this in the story I shared in chapter 1, in which the Feminist Icon seemed to see my interest in exiting, based on my own experience, as inherently flawed, when the care workers she knew were too busy working to *even entertain* the idea.

When I first conceptualized this project, a few care scholars and even the Carleton University research ethics committee advised me to redesign my project to focus on *working* care providers or people who rely on care – those they deemed most vulnerable. I nearly fell off my chair when the university ethics committee wrote to me saying that they thought the project was ethically sound, but that I should redesign my study *not* to examine privileged former care providers, but to centre the *most* vulnerable or *most* marginalized – that is, care recipients and care providers who are still doing the work. It was as if they somehow thought I hadn't thought of that as I wrote two comprehensive exams, a proposal, and the ethics application.

I also saw this common-sense assumption during my recruitment process, when some were quick to chime in that they didn't think a project on women "leaving" was relevant to the real struggles of real people. It was as if they thought issues of gender or intersectional equity somehow dissipate the moment someone gives their two weeks' notice or otherwise high-tails it out. When I distributed my recruitment poster, a researcher at a national care work union asked whether I'd consider interviewing marginalized people, indicating that my recruitment criteria of women who had stepped back from a caring role excluded them. Upon seeing my poster, another woman said, "Must be friggin' nice; I didn't bail on my kids." Others credited me for researching those in such "privileged" positions. The idea that it was a privilege to leave, or that only privileged women leave, was a refrain as I circulated the poster and told people about my study plans. Multiple people credited me for researching privilege, researching up, or researching those in power. This stood out, as I hadn't *once* been accused of researching privilege when I interviewed visual artists and public gallery curators as part of my master's research, but I received those comments on the regular with my focus on stepping back. It was pre-pandemic so perhaps how women live their lives wasn't on their radar, but still: *Had they truly not met anyone with an experience like the women in my study?*

In addition to making comments about my interest in privileged women, some suggested that I could do more to make my research more palatable. A colleague suggested that I should tell others that "the *only* reason I wanted to study the stories of former carers was to improve conditions of care and work for those currently in it." When I shared with Nora that there had been a bit of a "flinch factor" with my topic, she suggested that perhaps before I speak out about care workers experiencing harm or walking off the job, I could first begin by telling others that I am aware of power, privilege, and ableism. In my dissertation, I wrote about how she seemed to uphold dominant discourses of care in her advice to me, framing people who need care as the *most* vulnerable. I also suspect now that she was concerned about me. She too wanted to expand the conversation and stretch the stories we could tell about women's lives, but perhaps she didn't want me getting hurt or putting myself out for critique in the process.

But part of my politics was to be a bit unpalatable. Defiant. Tacky. Running counter. I must have commented to others dozens of times that I actually gave a shit about how women live their lives and didn't think it was always a privilege to exit or that only privileged women exit. I mean, is it really a privilege to not have the life you wanted, or to have to unravel the life you were building? To have to forfeit your wages and move in with a family for a couple years to physically and emotionally recover? As I fielded criticism, I also often told others that I didn't mind getting my hand slapped, that I was okay learning from some backlash. *I mean, I sort of was, I think?*

Continuing that disruptive work in this chapter, I examine women's stories of leaving, stepping back, or otherwise renegotiating responsibility for caring roles. I attend to tropes and the social functions that they serve – further revealing dominant relations and meanings of care, while nuancing some common-sense assumptions. This is not to say that my analysis challenges or disputes others' insights, as others are writing about care in different historical periods and contexts and taking aim at structural conditions. But women's counter stories do illustrate variations and shed light on how some experience leaving. Aiming to learn from their stories, I ask: What work is involved in getting out? How do women – *as political actors* – actively rethink, resist, and renegotiate dominant care-related expectations and meanings as part of a politics of responsibility? How do our conversations rearticulate meanings around care work and moral, feminine responsibility? I begin by analysing rhetorical conventions for speaking about leaving, move to considering how leaving has different stakes for different women (with some "flowing through" and others "wading through swamps"), and close by considering the culturally and politically significant work that women do to rethink, resist, or break down care-related expectations and meanings.

The analysis that I present in this chapter contributes to research and thinking on responsibility politics. Of note, Andrea Doucet (2022) develops a broad conception of responsibilities for care in her research on gendered divisions of household work and care. She distinguishes care tasks or activities of the "can you execute that?" variety from care responsibilities, which she argues are hard to measure on clock time. Folding laundry or making dinner are tasks that can be measured in discrete units of time, while "managing, organizing, and monitoring children's lives and activities" (449) are responsibilities that "can spread unpredictably across time" (450). In defining responsibilities, Doucet (2022) draws on Joan Tronto (2013), who notes that care processes involve noticing, taking responsibility, ensuring care needs get met or the work of caring is done, and observing or making judgments about what needs to change (see also Doucet and Klostermann 2023). Responsibilities go beyond time-bound tasks that can be observed and accomplished in the same room as someone (Doucet 2022). Such a robust conception of care-related responsibilities provides a strong incentive for looking across the life-course, as well as for looking at a wider range of care-negotiation strategies women use that extend beyond any particular care role or relationship.

With such a focus, I also draw inspiration from recent scholarship on responsibility politics. In their research on Swedish environmental movements, Håkan Thörn and Sebastian Svenberg (2016) develop the notion of a "politics of responsibility" to account for processes of responsibilization and de-responsibilization, as individuals both take responsibility for environmental causes (such as through expressing guilt or expressing individual moral agency), and resist or renegotiate responsibility (such as by redefining moral agency or calling on corporations or political institutions to take responsibility) (see also Klostermann 2023). They recognize "responsibilization as *a process involving negotiation and/or struggle*" (Thörn and Svenberg 2016, 595, emphasis in original).

Applying insights from their work, I orient to women as political actors engaged in a politics of responsibility, including when they contribute to conversations, which can be political spaces where women's interests or feminism(s) emerge (see Carrier-Moisan 2014). I explore in this chapter how much we can learn from women's political work. As I've argued elsewhere, care scholars at times maintain moral positions in expressing their desire to be able to care *more* or to provide relational care (such as in framing walking away or not taking individual responsibility for care as consistent with the logic of capitalist medicine) (see Klostermann 2023). Others argue that care workers themselves are uniquely positioned to "defend and promote caring as a central form of human practice" (Tronto 2020), but in this chapter I consider how we can learn more from care workers than that. One can of course respond "morally to others in the register of care" (Robinson 2019, 14), as a feminist ethic of care reminds us. Yet, as I illustrate, women's counter stories speak both to how providing care is *one of many ways* of offering a moral response or taking responsibility, and to how "our ways of responding morally are constructed in and through relationships and a wide variety of broad and specific contexts" (Robinson 2019, 17). Women's stories help in recasting care as a domain of struggle, with invitations for feminist theoretical care scholarship.

"Heartbreakers Leave" and Other Tropes

In speaking of care workers walking off the job after a COVID-19 outbreak at a Markham, Ontario, group home, Premier Doug Ford said, "What happened in Markham is heartbreaking. We just can't abandon the most vulnerable" (Delitala 2020). His comment is just one example of the moralizing language around stepping back from care that is also evident in media coverage promoting ideals of servitude, "heroine-ism," or feminine devotion. As the director of care at an Ontario nursing home said to me, "You can't instil empathy into a soul who doesn't have that sort of thing, but those people end up leaving" (Klostermann and Funk 2024, 208). In his view, the empathetic workers stay, which was a trope that stood out to me as I analysed rhetorical conventions in women's stories.

The common social expectation is that care workers "will work as long as it takes to get this work done" (Baines and Armstrong 2019, 9), and many workers themselves express a desire to "care more" (11). With dominant or disparaging views of people who need care (such as those framing them as a burden), women who leave are perhaps seen as (or see themselves as) contributing to the devaluation of those who need care. When care work is viewed as a gendered form of resistance, or a way to "contest uncaring management, governments and larger society" (Baines 2015, 205), it makes it hard to justify stepping back, as stepping back seems "uncaring" or like a way of devaluing the lives of people that one set out to value or "ought" to value.

The idea that "heartbreakers leave" is one trope that frames opting out of a caring role, or redistributing responsibility for care, as a self-ish, uncaring act. The term "heartbreaker" points straight to affective dimensions. It signals someone irresponsible in emotional relationships to the point of causing others distress. In our conversation, Julie, who was in her late twenties at the time we spoke, told the story of Joe, a person with an intellectual and developmental disability who she supported when she was a live-in assistant at L'Arche: "I was talking with Joe's stepdad, and I was like, 'I think I've finally tapped into Joe, like, I think we're finally friends!' And then his stepdad was like, "Yeah, until you leave him just like everyone else does. He's actually a smart guy, and he wasn't connecting with you because he was protecting himself.' I remember being like, Oh, my God! I'm one more person who's going to break his heart, and he just doesn't know that yet. He thinks that I'm probably in it for the long haul."

Julie differentiated heartbreakers who leave from those in it for the long haul, noting that Joe had been taught to close himself off or become more guarded with live-in assistants. Her story speaks to how understandings of care are handed to people in practice or in specific organizational contexts. While Julie recalled being touched by this conversation, to me it highlights how there were limited social scripts or rituals to support carers in that context in opting out of care responsibilities or in articulating their experiences in more complex ways, such as by exploring how they may also become attached or heartbroken themselves. There was no ritual closure. If we take women's stories of reaching their limits seriously, such an expectation – that good, moral women don't leave or that they should or might be in it for the long haul – is harmful for carers and those who need care alike. It keeps carers captive, limiting their agency and social mobility while making a claim on their lives and with care as a life sentence. Such a trope also positions care recipients as those "impacted," rather than as agentive subjects who might be able to negotiate or make meaning of such transitions. It makes leaving seem like a rare or unexpected occurrence, something to be let down by.

A related trope in the context of familial care was to frame stepping back or sharing responsibility as a way of "writing off" one's family members. That is also the kind of thing a heartbreaker does. In speaking of her family history, Gina talked about family members with mental health issues and noted that "back then" – decades ago – they wrote people off as "crazy" and sent them to the "loony bin" without more comprehensive understandings of "mental health issues" or supports for the "situational or social or what's going on in someone's life." As Gina said, "You were just written off." The idea here is that not providing care in one's family/home is a way of "writing off" a person. Such an ethical stance is informed by an awareness of the conditions of care in large-scale institutions. Yet it risks romanticizing the concept of home or home care supports (Chivers 2023). It also places the onus on individual family members to provide direct daily care indefinitely, and often without respite or the needed supports to pull it off. Such a trope relies on an "if not this, then that" logic – for instance, by idealizing intimate or familial care that is provided by women, rather than pushing for public supports for communal or congregate care. The idea that not providing direct daily care *for* a person is a way of not caring *about* a person (Davidson 2015) was visible in women's stories of placing their relatives in institutional care, as well as in critiques they faced for doing so. Anne recalled one journalist referring to her as "selfish" and as a "line jumper" when she dropped her son off at developmental services (after no longer being able to provide care at home).

Taken together, the tropes presented above – that it is uncaring or emotionally reckless to leave – make up and are backed by dominant circulating narratives that frame care-related responsibilities as the individual responsibility of individual workers or individual family members. Across Canada, with so much political focus on recruiting and retaining women in care work, it's notable that women "leaving care," in some contexts, is not institutionally recognized or supported. There are no handbooks on "how to leave," nor are there enough circulating stories to help people who provide and rely on care to understand the value of leaving or to access the needed conceptual resources to talk about or reconcile their life experiences.

There are limited supports for those who want to exit, despite the fact that a fuller understanding – not just of care equity but of gender equity – seems to encourage just that.

In looking at these tropes, we can see how one's ability to step back or share responsibility with others, as well as one's ability to lean on or access private- or public-sector supports (such as respite, home care, or residential care options) shapes one's "choices" and the stories one tells. It is these conditions that give rise to moral demands for women not to "break hearts" or "dump others," or face the costs or consequences of doing so.

Yet we also know that women *do* leave, step back, or share responsibility all the time and across their lives. They find ways to circumvent, exit, or step away from care.

Women Leave: Finding Flow or Wading through Swamps

In a study of how social inequalities mediate workplace change, Janet Siltanen and colleagues (2009) distinguish between those who "flow through" such changes and others who get "swamped" or need to engage in "comparatively more belaboured" work to navigate workplace change (1016). While some stories of stepping back from a caring role seemed easy to reconcile or "flow through," others were more like wading through swamps and involved an incredible range of belaboured and ongoing work, including in relation to one's sense of self and self-expectations.

Finding "flow" and summing their story up quickly, Troy recalled high-tailing it off to university when the time came, saying, "I left town as quickly as possible when I turned eighteen. My younger sister had to pick up the slack of caring for the kids [in my mom's home day care]." To give another example, Marilyn, a retired nurse and former family caregiver who was born in the late 1940s and was around age seventy at the time of meeting, talked about turning down requests to care for her mother-in-law when her own children were young. As Marilyn put it, "I backed out of that one pretty quick! I was not about to become her maid." Vicki, an AIDS activist in her sixties, also told a story of hitting the brakes on a care gig. She was out for dinner with a woman she supported and set limits on the support she could provide right then and there: "I told her that her anger toward me was something I needed changed in order for me to continue supporting her [as part of her care team], and everything ground to a halt." Neither of them stuck around to order dessert. Rhonda, a former mental health nurse in her seventies, remembered that when she was about ready to retire, she shoved a note under her boss's door that just said "bye." Her co-worker said, "You have to give your two weeks' notice," to which Rhonda quipped, "So fire me." These stories of stepping back seemed fun and easy to tell. There were no back stories or elaborate explanations. I didn't pick up on any guilt, shame, or regret. For some people in some situations, stepping back or setting limits was just part of life. In fact, when Anne talked about that journalist who called her "selfish," she didn't exactly seem bogged down by the weight of the moral scrutiny. With a deadpan delivery, Anne said, "You know, she's really entitled to her opinion." She had a nonchalant and unfazed presentation of self. She was aware of the social expectations to care but had agency in negotiating them. As her story shows, with sufficient conceptual resources or justifications to draw on, leaving or setting limits can be easier to talk about or "flow through."

Yet, others told stories about struggling to move on or still feeling stuck years later, with accounts that challenge the idea that leaving was even remotely a privilege. Paid and unpaid family carers alike underscored that there can be real costs and consequences to leaving, with women who leave paying the price. Carrie said, "You have to go through fire. Get shunned first. You get hated on … Everybody and the cat is going to talk bad about you … That's the price to pay to get out from being their caregiver." Speaking to the social costs of setting limits on the support she could provide to family members, Carrie said that she felt as though she had been kicked out of the community, left out of intimate family happenings, such as the opportunity to feel her pregnant sister's stomach when her baby kicked.

Offering another example of the costs and consequences of leaving care, Julie talked about her grandmother's cousin who had devoted her life to service and caring for others as a nun, only to be left "essentially homeless" when she left the convent. In unpacking this, Julie stated that she herself had been "fine financially" while in a live-in care worker position but was "faced with this harsh reality of financial burden, after having dedicated [her] life – a year of [her] life – to something." In addition to stories about women being socially shunned or struggling financially, we also saw multiple examples of women's health issues, as explored in chapter 4. Nora, for instance, said it well when she joked that she wished that she would have been able to leave her job at the residential group home with her "health intact" and her "sanity intact." She also spoke to the lack of support that had come her way, saying, "Like, how come I didn't get a fucking goodbye party? Or like a card?" We both laughed at that, and laughed even harder when she admitted that she hadn't been well enough to work, let alone to wave her little hat around at a party. A card would have been nice, though!

Having looked at women's stories, and reflected on the stakes of them, we'll explore below the work involved in renegotiating responsibility for care.

The Strategies Women Use to "Get Out" Tell Us What They Are Up Against

In leaving caring roles or renegotiating care-related responsibilities, the women in this study put work into: (1) negotiating their own and others' care needs in the face of ongoing demands to care; (2) reorienting to their sense of selves; (3) rethinking relations and meanings of care (including gendered, moral imperatives to care); and (4) imagining alternatives for their lives. The stories they told, and the strategies they used, teach us about what they were up against. They speak to how care is socially and culturally constructed, with gendered power relations extending beyond any one role. We can see in some of the following stories how caring can provide a sense of self, self-worth, or identity as a "good" person (Day 2013; Funk and Outcalt 2019), especially for women who are socialized to "fulfil a vision of ourselves as good only when we attend to the needs of others" (Kittay 1999, 24). We can also see how women find ways to challenge neoliberal agendas that assign individual responsibility and ways to rethink dominant ideas about care being an "important obligation for women," which are ideas rooted in "a moral division of labour" (Folbre et al. 2021, 175).

Notably, women's stories and strategies show traces of the conceptual resources or supports they had access to that can aid in moving in a different direction or framing things in a different way. Regarding the conceptual resources or supports needed to loosen the ties that bind, it stood out that Gina was making sense of her life situation in conversation with other grandmothers, while Julie referenced scholarly or political teachings she had come across in university. In different contexts and with different levels of access to conceptual resources, they were finding ways to release themselves from projects they had previously committed to. Their stories speak to the need for expanding and stretching circulating narratives of care to support women in imagining and living out other possibilities.

Negotiating One's Own and Others' Care Needs

As political actors engaged in a politics of responsibility, the women I interviewed put thought into reorienting to their own and others' care needs, including as they arranged for others to provide support in their absence. For some, stepping back meant having to release themselves from the weight of the expectations to provide direct care and from the responsibilities they had previously taken on. Around the time Troy resigned, they remembered asking themselves, "Is this fair to be around people when I feel like I can't even take care of myself?" This question is one example of the moral negotiating that takes place, as people rethink how care could be reorganized and reassigned. In the stories they told, Troy seemed to be trying to convince themselves that it was okay to leave, and finding ways to comfort themselves by thinking the people they had supported will "figure it out," that they "know what's going on in their own lives," that Troy didn't "have to be responsible for that." As Troy said, "Ever since I started being off [work], I'm like, my clients survived without me, they will continue to survive without me, other people will do this work. It's okay; I need to take care of myself." In the face of dominant ideals about heartbreakers leaving, Troy framed leaving a paid care work role as in the best interests of others. Importantly, they also recognized their embeddedness in more extended relationships, articulating a collective understanding of care that went well beyond one individual pinkie swearing to serve others indefinitely.

Others also talked about engaging in work to care for themselves or to recover physically and mentally after leaving. Gina, a family carer, said, "You have to start thinking about yourself and start going back to the doctor and getting your heath taken care of and getting yourself where you used to be." In speaking of moving out of her mom's apartment, she said, "The first night [home], I couldn't sleep, because I was so used to listening to her breathing. You would have thought I would come home and pass out, but I didn't. I was still on the caregiver time warp." Gina recalled thinking, "Where is she? Why can't I hear her?" She also recalled that it "took three months to get back" to being able to sleep without "waking up listening for her breathing." Her description of resetting her body after care speaks to how she had embodied the relationship, as well as to how the experience had impacted her.

Paid care workers also talked about (the belaboured work of) listening to their bodies, attending medical or physio appointments, accepting care from others, slowing down their everyday routines, and processing their experiences in therapy or with friends. Carrie said, "I worked on my mental health, developed my self-worth, started noticing toxicity in relationships." For some, leaving also involved figuring out housing, income, and social assistance. Carrie relinquished her vehicle and started growing her own food to save money, while Nora gave up her housing, exited the workforce, and moved in with her mom to spend a couple of years recovering, with wage penalties to boot. Nora said that when you're "go go going and you're not listening to your body, you're not listening to this, and you're not listening to that, as soon as you stop, it all kind of comes out." With real work involved, Troy found another roommate to "reduce [their] costs," and jumped through hoops to apply for social assistance, including workers' compensation, employment insurance, and long-term disability. All these activities speak to the limited worker protections, buffers, or supports they had. While support never fully disappeared for the women I interviewed, and most had a social safety net to fall back on, we can see in their stories how depleting their experiences were, and how much work was involved in renegotiating responsibilities for care, including responsibilities to care for themselves.

With care as a domain of struggle, some told stories of setting limits or stepping back from care in one context only to be launched into another care role or live out "care dynamics" in other ways. At the time of speaking to me, many were still navigating ongoing care relationships and expectations that extended beyond any one role. Demands to care for others seemed like part of the price of living in a society with inadequate public-sector supports for people with real care needs, which at times called for some drastic measures.

In our conversation together, Carrie said, "*Even now*, I'm still unravelling the ways where I respond to others before myself … It's this constant, like I said, always measuring and reflecting, because, you know, it's so easy to go back to being a doormat … *Even now*, I'd drop everything and run, I have to watch that." Replete with the phrase "even now," which is a statement about time, Carrie called attention to the range of work involved in renegotiating responsibility for care, long after leaving. For her, stepping back wasn't as simple as resigning from the work or saying no to shifts. There was no "clean break." She also talked about a family member who had "worked, *had to work*, so hard to get out from under the care of others – to get out from under caring for others." She made important points in calling attention to the range of work involved and to power relations that, in some care contexts, can position carers "under" others.

At the time of speaking, Troy said they were staying vigilant and trying to notice when they had "urges" to care, as it felt like an "unhealthy relationship" or "addiction" they were recovering from. They joked that they were trying to stop themselves from yelling "I'll go with you!" when others ask them to help or to accompany them to medical appointments. Cheering at Troy's comment, I said to them, "I resonate with stepping back from one organization or feeling like it's a clean break and then still having all these kinds of caregiving dynamics in other areas, you know? It's hard to shake." Relatedly, Gina laughed when mentioning that she sold her car so she wouldn't have to be on call to run errands for her mother. "Yeah, yeah! I'm glad you got rid of the car," I cheered. But it was clear that "stepping back" took more than moving out of her mother's place or selling the car, as she was still negotiating demands to coordinate aspects of her mother's care, including by scheduling and overseeing all her appointments.

In the context of inadequate public services, and against the backdrop of pervasive cultural imperatives, "opportunities" to care extend beyond any particular role or relationship. Care is a domain of struggle. As we've explored, women's stories weren't of taking "uncaring" counter paths per se. The paths some women found didn't run counter, as they were still hooked in relationships, still facing demands to care, and still working out how to live alongside others or make sense of what they owed others. There was no escape and nowhere to go. That said, while it may not always be possible to separate or untether, we can see in women's stories the importance of expanding imaginaries of care, to help create the conditions to be able to do so.

Rethinking and Challenging Moral, Gendered Imperatives to Care

The women in this study put time and effort into actively rethinking meanings of care, including by challenging moral, gendered imperatives or rethinking their sense of selves and self-expectations. They were political actors "creating meanings and critique alongside and with me" (Carrier-Moisan as quoted by Cole et al. 2014, 144). "There's something there that needs to be unpacked," Troy said with enthusiasm, as we talked about the phrase "I couldn't do your job," which was a "compliment" they too had often received as a paid care worker. With that being one of several examples of things that needed unpacking, participants in this study were actively interrogating their care histories, and at times even redefining what care meant to them.

This was part of the work of "loosening the grip," with participants telling "stories that have the potential to expand dominant social imaginaries of caregiving" (Sawchuk et al. 2024, 329). Taken together, they broke down dominant, hegemonic meanings of care, lessening the stronghold of moralized ideologies, while challenging neoliberal agendas that assign responsibility at the individual level. To do so, they needed to be able to access conceptual resources and circulating narratives that supported them in resituating or recontextualizing their stories.

At the time of speaking, Carrie was still putting energy into processing her experience of resigning from paid care work and setting limits on the family care she could provide to her siblings. She said, "It's just always ongoing work to define caregiving and make sure it's not sacrificial." She too spoke of staying vigilant. She also talked about trying to reconcile her own need to step back with her belief in "intergenerational care," which was important to her as an Indigenous woman. While she valued practices of living "communally," and saw the importance of tenets to "stick together," she was also actively rethinking what she herself had the capacity to do. Stepping back was something Carrie still wrestled with, as she was trying to distance herself from her past identification as a care provider, which had been a primary sense of self-worth. In a playfully self-deprecating way, Carrie poked fun at her historical self, who *used to* find caring meaningful or who *used to* love supporting people "in the fire." She said "in the fire" as though to sound pretentious or "hoity-toity," or to suggest that caring *used to* be something she would brag about. She also self-deprecatingly recalled that if she was "experiencing distress or conflict," it was easier for her to say, "Oh, forget about that! How are *you*? Oh, you don't have enough groceries for a week?" or "*Oh*, I can get him jeans that'll fit. Don't worry!" She dramatically re-enacted forfeiting her own needs, in a way that seemed to help put some distance between her past and current self.

With her artistic impulses as a storyteller, Carrie delivered her life story in a comic mode and was at ease challenging "familiar meanings and [putting herself] at the mercy of the situation" (Hendriks 2012, 459). Humour seemed to offer a way to loosen the grip of expectations to care for others against all odds. Just as a comic frame "allows the most rigid societies to creatively stretch their frameworks and to play with their presumed identities" (Lewis 2007, 52), Carrie used humour to challenge dominant frames of reference and to break down moralizing expectations to care for others that she had previously adhered to.

Laughing as she spoke, Carrie said, "Some pedophiles groom children for that abuse; my mother groomed me to be a caregiver for my sister." She recalled providing direct daily care from age two onwards and cited her family's financial struggles and her mother's mental health issues. As if delivering a joke, she said, "I was two years old, and I did all [my sister's] feeding. My mother says she couldn't – that she only knew that my sister's diaper was dirty because I told her ... From a small, small age, my mom would talk about how I knew what my sister wanted before anybody else did. *Some magical intuition!*" Carrie framed her past care experiences as ridiculous, absurd, or something to make light of, which seemed to offer a way to challenge those conditions, while releasing herself from care-related responsibilities that had been debilitating. If it had been a bit of a joke, not a serious, sanctimonious life path, perhaps it was okay to step back. Further, in emphasizing the abject and detailing her denigration, Carrie pushed against those dominant, hegemonic understandings of care that had previously had her by the neck.

Nora also engaged in work to challenge normative expectations around care. "I've thought about it so much over the years and have talked about it so much too," Nora said. She too was actively processing her experience, with statements like "I didn't have any sort of closure" or "I still struggle with the whole care thing," offering examples of what I mean. Nora expressed that resigning from her work at the group home had had her rethinking her sense of self and self-expectations. As she recalled, "I still felt so guilty and so tied to it ... [Even after leaving,] I didn't really know who I was without it." What was at stake in Nora's story seemed to be who she was as a person. "Well, who am I then? Who am I?" she asked. While there were practical considerations to leaving, it also involved work to reorient to her sense of self and self-expectations. When caring is so deeply ingrained, expected, and self-defining, and when it provides a sense of self, self-worth, or identity as a "good" person, it takes hard work to loosen gendered, moral ideals of care (that can feel like chains around one's heart) and to create a new sense of self or meaning.

Similar to the work Carrie did above, Nora also put work into reconceptualizing meanings of care. "I don't know if it's caring itself that's the problem," she said. "I mean, I think caring and caregiving is something that's so integral to life, like we all need it, you know? ... And it's one of those, 'Oh, if we all cared for each other more, life would be better.' But at the same time, [caring for others can be] really unhealthy and really controlling and really traumatic and really just debilitating." In a way that I think is instructive, Nora wrestled with dominant conceptions of care. I appreciate that she didn't land on a firm answer but modelled a way of thinking things through, attending to contradictions. With a "but at the same time," Nora hedged, making space for other points of emphasis. She underscored that care is important, but also hinted that moral imperatives to care shouldn't come at such a price for individual women. As a political actor engaged in a politics of responsibility, her account highlights how the making of a caring world goes beyond "all car[ing] for each other more" and involves sharing responsibilities or letting women leave as necessary.

Gina also put work into rethinking her relationship to care or what she owed others. As explored in chapter 4, no longer having "what it took" was a tough pill to swallow, as she had attached moral value to caring as something she was supposed to want, and as something she saw as part of her job as a grandmother. Yet she certainly wasn't getting a "pass" from caregiving, stiffing others with the work. Gina mentioned that she no longer had the patience, capacity, or interest in taking care of her granddaughter, but also shared a story about how much thought she put into helping others step in. At a recent pool party, she had set out some craft supplies for the child to "let her mom and dad do the crafts and stuff with her." Making sense of this, Gina said that the "old Gina" would have been right down on the floor, hanging out with the child for the whole party, but she no longer had what it took. She said, "I cannot give the proper care ... I'm literally, like I said, burnt out. I can't do it. Maybe a few years down the road. I've never stopped caring for people; I just can't do it 24/7." Gina put effort into rethinking dominant moral imperatives to care for others. It stood out to me that she distinguished between "caring for people" and "giv[ing] the proper care," and that she set some temporal limits in saying that she couldn't do it "24/7" or "these days." She seemed to articulate a collective understanding of "care" that goes beyond providing it indefinitely.

Julie also put thought into confronting dominant, hegemonic under standings of care, in making sense of leaving. In speaking of resigning from L'Arche, she said, "I really value [the work of direct care], but it doesn't mean that I want to be involved in it." Hers was a simple, yet powerful, statement. She planted her feet – stating that she values caring – before pushing off – noting that she personally doesn't want to be involved. In a way, she seemed to align with feminist scholars who recognize care's importance, but she also drew a boundary on such an invitation, as it applied to her personally or as an individual. "Oh, yeah, cool," I said to Julie in response. "It's powerful to hear you valuing the work, but almost wanting to say more with your life than just meeting someone's everyday needs."

Given that there are no handbooks on "how to leave" and that dominant circulating narratives provide limited support for women to negotiate hazardous or inequitable circumstances, finding some ways to rethink and reframe gendered assumptions and expectations around care is part of what it takes for some to "flow through."

Imagining Alternatives for One's Life and Work

Women's choices are also shaped by the possibilities we can imagine for ourselves. Wendy Luttrell (2020) writes, "Decades of research has established that social inequalities, especially related to class, race, and gender, shape how people learn what they feel entitled to, constrained by, and how they envision their future possibilities" (6). For women in this study, part of the work of "loosening the grip" involved imagining other possibilities for their lives. Their stories helped me to think about how improving care conditions isn't just a matter of ensuring better supports for those in caring roles, but ensuring they have other avenues for self-worth or other possibilities or pathways to try out. So much resides in the imagination.

In speaking of resigning from paid care work, Troy brought an important trans lens to the issue, which gave them tools and a lot of traction with unpacking normative gender expectations to care. In speaking of caring for others, Troy explained, "It's so ingrained in my identity and my career, and I'm really scared if I step away from it completely. Like, what does that mean, like, how do I identify? ... What type of person does it make me?" Like Nora, Troy mentioned how care work had meant something; it had been a way to carve out an unconventional, queer life path that went beyond professional work or family-making. They couldn't see themselves in a board room or an industry job, and they had never felt so embraced in life as they had been in the care sector. Care just felt like home, which they noted also made it hard to imagine another life path. So, beyond improving conditions of work and care on the clock, their story spoke to the need for expanding paths for women and LGBTQ groups to ensure they can imagine other possibilities for their lives.

Indeed, the hazards of contemporary life that participants pointed to, *and had analyses of*, went beyond the work. Troy identified other "structural things in [their] day" that shaped and constrained their options, such as "all the transphobia and homophobia and sexism and … poverty [and] ridiculous student loans." They recounted being misgendered and concerned for their physical safety when harassed by strangers threatening to throw them in front of the bus. Their problem wasn't just about work/organizational conditions. As Troy said, "I don't think any of that stuff has ever been taken into consideration. It's like, 'Oh you just didn't do enough self-care.'" Further illustrating how more extended conditions matter, Carrie stated that she had been exhausted from everything she "navigated from being a homeless kid or, before that, a kid living at home with parents who didn't care." The life-spanning relations of participants' lives were part of the story and part of what variously made it hard to leave or hard to find their footing afterwards. It's not just about working conditions in a particular care work role, but about improving conditions of care, work, and life. These are matters of gender and intersectional equity.

Vicki, a long-time AIDS activist, also spoke to the need for other paths or places to which one can retreat. Speaking as a woman in her sixties who didn't have kids, she said, "There's no place for me to retreat to, right? Others can retreat behind an appearance of heterosexuality and child-raising and family life, right? But, for me, that's not possible." We also explored this further.

> VICKI: It's also [interesting] if you – if you as an adult … don't necessarily fit into [those] social narratives about caring, like, you know, parenting or mothering or whatever. You kind of have to make it up, right?
> JANNA: Oh, yeah, rather than wedging into this "good mother" or good –
> VICKI: You know, there's no mother. There's no – I'm not a mother. So, it's, like, you have to do it some other way if you're gonna do it, you know? Or you have to call it by some other name if you're gonna call it, you know?

There's no one way, or right way, to interpret this, and I'm not even sure I'm seeing the full picture, but I think Vicki's point about having to find alternative ways of living or imagining one's life is an important one. Similar to what Troy had to say, Vicki highlighted the importance of expanding paths for women and queer people and ensuring they can imagine other possibilities for their lives, which, I've come to appreciate, is work that can happen in conversation.

Nearing the end of our conversation together, I shared with Nora that I had been questioning whether I could stop first telling people how good and well-meaning I had been when I first started as a care worker, before mentioning that I burnt out and had to resign. I also said that I had been wondering if the more that I moralized or idealized my entrance into care, the further I had to fall off the "care cliff" by in turn framing it as a violation and betrayal. It seemed like an *aha* moment for Nora as well, as she said, "I think that I can let go of that idealized version of myself – untangle myself from that romanticized version of it." *Aha.* "I think that I can let go" is how she put it. Together we reached for new meanings, expanding our narrative range.

It was at the end of a long three-hour conversation with Carrie, just before I turned the recorder off, that she shared that she had been working on her mental health, accepting care from others, and building a network of support. We both seemed to challenge the idea that women should constantly be of use or of service to justify breathing, and I said to Carrie, "Okay, maybe that's what that is, maybe we don't have to carry it. Maybe we don't have to …" Carrie paused before smiling and saying, "That's kind of the worst too, after all that fronting, and you're like *awwwwwhh*." She laughed and sighed a full-body exhale. That *awwwwwhh* seemed to be a way of saying that maybe we didn't have to care for others at the expense of ourselves, and maybe we didn't have to keep ruminating, as there were other, alternative ways to craft our lives. Such an example is a testament to "women's sociality as imperative to the survival and development of feminism" (Taylor 2008, 720). Sometimes we get somewhere.

Rethinking Care as a Domain of Struggle

Above I laid out some of the dominant, hegemonic assumptions around leaving care that position women who leave as selfish, emotionally reckless, and privileged. While some experiences of stepping back seem easier to reconcile, others involved belaboured work and certainly weren't a "privilege." We also see in women's counter stories how they actively negotiate these dominant understandings, while also renegotiating responsibilities for care and repositioning themselves in moral, gendered relations. Women borrow from inherited narratives and revise and recast them too.

As political actors actively engaged in a politics of responsibility (Thörn and Svenberg 2016; see also Klostermann 2023), these women were actively finding ways to resist, rethink, and renegotiate their situations. As we explored, for some in some situations, stepping back doesn't simply involve packing one's bags, resigning from a job, or walking away when you can. Selling your vehicle doesn't cut it either. We can see how much time and work can go into negotiating one's own and others' needs, rethinking one's sense of self, redefining care work, and imagining possibilities. For some, it takes an incredible amount of effort to loosen the grip of care-related expectations, rethinking one's referential relationships to oneself, to others, and to care. As illustrated, these relational care-negotiation processes can involve multiple layers of interpretive intra-subjective work. These weren't stories of women wanting to care more/indefinitely. Nor were they stories of women "leaving when they can," getting a "pass" from caring for others, enacting privileged irresponsibility, or deputizing care to others. Instead, we can see the need for countering assumptions about exiting being a matter of privilege and status that some (fetishized caregiver victims) couldn't even imagine.

The strategies explored in this chapter tell us about gendered power relations that extend beyond any one paid or unpaid care work role. They speak to the need for more expansive circulating narratives that help ensure women have other legitimate ways to frame their lives and imagine possibilities. Just as some joke that you don't know how married you are until you get divorced, the same goes for care: you don't know how far in it you are until you go to leave. That isn't to say that everyone is in as far, but that one's strategies for extricating oneself or loosening the ties that bind can teach us about the project one has been handed, as well as about the conditions of one's life.

Another contribution in this chapter was theorizing care as a domain of struggle. Past studies on nursing and teaching have found that some leave helping professions due to moral distress, with some even leaving to preserve their sense of moral integrity or moral self-conceptions (Corley et al. 2005; Kelly 1998; Santoro 2018). We saw that when Troy talked about not wanting to be the "worker no one wants." Further, my findings illustrate how some women are *still* implicated and *still* actively engaged in making up their lives in relation to "care" long after "leaving." It's worth considering whether newspaper headlines about a so-called mass exodus of care workers underestimate the *ongoing* work involved or the ways in which some are still caught up in care as a domain of struggle, in a broader politics of responsibility, long after. It strikes me that most reporting on the issue of workers' leaving focuses on the unmet needs of patients or on issues of work overload or "burn-out," without a recognition of how hard or disruptive such transitions can be for those making them. Limited attention has been paid to former care workers' struggles, let alone their insights. I'm not aware of any "veterans of care" support groups or collective spaces for women to process or heal, although a fuller understanding, not just of care equity but of gender equity, seems to invite that. I don't know: Is it worth creating some space for collective mourning for women whose lives have been upended, or who are still working through it? Would it be worth hosting a Care Junkie Recovery Group to bring other grieving women together?

Extending Andrea Doucet's (2021) point that care responsibilities are hard to measure on clock time, as they aren't just tasks that can be observed and accomplished in a room (see also Tronto 2013), we can see in this chapter how care responsibilities extend beyond any particular care relationship. Cultural imperatives to care reach into and across our lives, shaping our relationships with our sense of selves, self-understandings, and stories. They extend across time and space and beyond any one role or responsibility. Care is always contested, always negotiated. Care is a domain of struggle.

What I think is striking is that women in this study weren't simply restating the importance of care or reiterating how people deserve to have their care needs met or how care isn't valued and should be. They didn't simply highlight how care is socially necessary work that needs to be provided and supported politically. Nor did they simply argue that carers deserve to have their care needs met, or that we need to "care for the carer." What we can most learn from them isn't that "care matters" or care needs to be defended and promoted as a central human practice. They say more than that.

As moral meaning-makers (Eicher-Catt 2005), the women in this study were actively unpacking and rethinking moralized conceptions of care at the individual level, highlighting the need for exits and off-ramps. Their stories are testaments to how the making of a caring world goes beyond "all car[ing] for each other more," and requires limits and boundaries as well as options to exit or share responsibility. Individualizing understandings of care need to be rethought. Women's stories underscore that we need to value, invest in, and otherwise improve care, *and* need to ensure women have other worthwhile, legitimate ways to make a life or make something of themselves. Women and girls need liveable story structures. Gendered power relations and dominant imaginaries of care – that construct our worth or non-worth and shape our sense of what's possible – are part of the story.

Final Thoughts

This chapter brings into view the stories women tell, and the strategies they use, to rethink and release themselves from moral, gendered expectations to care. We looked at some dominant tropes used to talk about women leaving, at differences in whether women "find flow" or "wade through swamps" in telling their stories, and at strategies women use to release the ties that bind them to care work.

Moving beyond a focus on broader structural dynamics or patterns, this chapter challenges common-sense assumptions that women just want to care more, and that leaving is a matter of status and privilege. Looking at the constructedness of people's stories, and at counter stories in particular, tells a different story.

As political actors, the women in this study were broadening their understandings of care. It strikes me how much effort and thought they put into redefining care, rethinking who is worthy of care, and rethinking – or lessening the stronghold of – moralized or individualized understandings. It wasn't just that they needed to leave or say no, but that they needed ways to do so without feeling like immoral subjects failing at femininity. They were actively rethinking dominant assumptions, expectations, and meanings around care, framing their experiences in ways that allowed for some limits, boundaries, or counter paths. As illustrated, women find very different strategies for leaving (depending on circumstances, resources, narratives they have access to), which also raises further questions about the contexts they are in or the ways they are "set up," which is the focus of chapter 6.

In the next chapter, we'll examine patterns and contradictions in how women in different age cohorts and contexts are summoned into caring roles across the life-course and with differences in self/other care relationships or in their self-expectations. We'll take a closer look at "normative expectations that are institutionalized through structures" (Grenier et al. 2020, 22), considering how women in different social locations came to inhabit, make sense of, and negotiate a range of caring subject positions in Ontario's care economy. *But, first, a quick interlude ...*

Interlude: A Different Kind of #MeToo?

In 2020, when news broke of the sex abuse scandal involving L'Arche founder Jean Vanier, I felt like I could finally take the duct tape off my mouth, after years of flinching when people described him as a living saint or L'Arche as heaven on Earth. In a L'Arche International internal inquiry into the abuse, Vanier was described as initiating manipulative and coercive sex with multiple women. One witness recalled Vanier saying to her, "This is not us, this is Mary and Jesus. You are chosen, you are special, this is secret." Another witness testified that she "wrote to Jean Vanier to say that it was unbearable what he had done," and that he responded by simply saying that he thought the letter was good. He positioned her as desperate for his approval.

In response to the scandal, public accounts wrestled with the downfall of a charismatic spiritual leader or rushed to distinguish the good, moral work of L'Arche communities worldwide from Vanier's dirty doings. I felt sick that in some opinion pieces the writers seemed to express relief that the people who were sexually abused were care workers, not people with developmental disabilities. They seemed to be okay with a version of "community" in which only some get raped, with lines around who is worthy of care. As I read through responses to the news, I did not see a single article, or a single sentence in any of the articles I read, that considered how the institutionalized structures at L'Arche had set the stage for the exploitation and abuse of women. There wasn't a whiff about gendered power structures that promote feminine servitude in the context of care. There was nothing exploring care as a form of gender-based structural violence (see Streeter 2024).

When I wrote a short op-ed (Klostermann 2020), I truly felt like I was taking the duct tape off my mouth as I called attention to how Vanier's abusive approach had informed the organizational culture at L'Arche. I mentioned the conditions of extreme overwork, as well as how spiritual and emotional manipulation had been part of the job. I shared how L'Arche assistants were coached in submissiveness, coaxed to forfeit our power, and cued to say that we got more than we gave. I took aim at how elite L'Arche leaders were set apart from a feminized workforce composed of young, working-class, racialized, and migrant workers. I also shared about my own struggles, writing, "I feel sick that L'Arche exploited my desire to be good, blamed me for burning out, and denied my request to reduce my hours when I hit an emotional breaking point." I presented a feminist argument about the degrada-tion of women in an organization that spiritualizes sexism and debases women's work. When the desk editor at the *Toronto Star* assigned it the headline "L'Arche International Has a History of Exploiting Women," I felt like the tape was off my mouth.

I also felt the stakes of this. The night before the op-ed was published, I worried that by speaking out, I would be transgressing social mandates for women to be good or not upset anyone – that I'd be kicked out of the club. What club, I don't know, but I was at a building stage of my life, and this felt like a big risk. I worried that my perspective was too provocative or that others, including future hiring committee members, might see that I wasn't a happy-go-lucky good girl. Chris Kraus (2006) asks, "Why does everyone think women are debasing themselves when we expose the con-ditions of our own debasement?" (211), and I think that was part of it too.

I commented to my PhD supervisor, Susan, that I felt like I would be getting myself into trouble with the op-ed, that I should have learned my lesson from that UK conference. "I mean, is it that I can't help myself? That I'm a glutton for punishment?" I couldn't understand why I was making life harder for myself than it needed to be. "But you," Susan said warmly, "you like taking chances. You like taking on challenges even when they make your knees shake and you don't know how they'll turn out." It was true, I did. I had to admit there was plea-sure in testing things out, learning from the response. Like a stand-up comic who learns from the laugh of the crowd, I was learning from the knee-jerk responses of myself and others.

And, although I readied myself to get my hand slapped when the op-ed went live, what happened from there surprised me. I heard from L'Arche assistants around the world and from other family caregivers and paid care workers who resonated with my words. Several expressed that it gave them a way to talk about things, that there was power and truth to it. One L'Arche assistant mentioned that she read it dozens of times and even met with her housemates to discuss it. Their responses seemed like ways they were saying "me too" or "I'm with ya, girl." With each email or direct message that I received, I felt less alone. I could see I was part of a bigger group of women fighting back.

It seemed, to me, like a different kind of #MeToo.[1] I certainly didn't want to conflate or essentialize women's struggles as care workers with sexual assault, but the work we were doing felt important. We were speaking truth to silence, speaking up against women's subordination in caring roles, and claiming solidarity with one another. We were challenging the idea that women's liberation had already been achieved (or nearly) with laws that support gender equity, by calling attention to inequities that had been overlooked. We were addressing the ways we had been made vulnerable or set up for intimate losses.

Yet it wasn't a different kind of #MeToo. It really wasn't.

I'm not trying to dwell on the negative, but for every encounter or conversation I had about care work that just felt like wildfire or had that disruptive, emancipatory potential, there was another one that puttered along or fizzled out. At times it felt like the person I was speaking to just wasn't getting it or getting me. Even during my research, while I thought of myself as hosting a "Care Junkie Recovery Group" with each interview I conducted, that wasn't what some had signed up for or were even remotely interested in. Not everyone had been brought to their knees as a care worker or left struggling to escape an abusive situation. Not everyone was pissed off about the same things. As much as I wanted to edge in with grand sweeping statements about "reaching the limits of the care economy," about the "shit society throws at women," or about "expectations for women to care against all odds and at the expense of ourselves and regardless of conditions," that was hard to do given how much context matters. As some women I interviewed would have me know, it wasn't *all* women. Some of my punchy turns of phrase – whether in writing or in conversation – just didn't fly. It was hard to speak in the "we" or to essentialize or conflate *all* women or *all* care work. There was no universal, ahistorical, apolitical story.

This all came with the invitation for me to dig a bit deeper and work a bit harder to understand how context matters. The next chapter does just that.

---

1 In 2017, a few days after the news about Harvey Weinstein's sexual harassment broke in the *New York Times*, the hashtag "#MeToo" went viral on Twitter when actress Alyssa Milano tweeted, "If you've been sexually harassed or assaulted write 'me too' as a reply to this tweet." Her tweet helped to popularize #MeToo, which was a term coined by Tarana Burke in 2006, as part of a grassroots initiative to speak out against sexual violence against young Black women and girls. In the United States, Canada, and beyond, the #MeToo movement has drawn critical attention to the extent of women's experiences of sexual assault or harassment. It cleared space for women to access services and gave more voice and visibility to their struggles.

Chapter Six

Thinking "Differently and More Deeply about Care Stories": Women "Set Up" and Summoned across the Life-Course

My Mom started this thing with my brother, because she would only ever have twenty bucks for back-to-school clothes for him, which, I mean, you can't even get a pair of running shoes at Walmart for twenty bucks. She would go on and on about how he would only buy clothes with me. "Well, I try to take him shopping Carrie, he won't buy anything." Well, for twenty bucks, what do you expect? But I had grown up like that. Back when Value Village was actually a cheaper option [laughs]. Now, it's like I may as well go to Walmart [laughs]. So, I would go, "*Ohh*, only I connect with my brother." She would exploit my wanting to be connected. I'd take my brother shopping for a whole weekend to all these discount places and we'd find him cool clothes that he was okay with. We found cool jeans – I'd find them for six dollars apiece and I'd probably kick in about fifty dollars of my own money, because I didn't want him to go through what I went through.

– Carrie

In the explication above, Carrie expressed that her moral desire to connect with and support her brother had been exploited in a context of material disadvantage. She also remembered that she had thought, "*Ohh*, only I connect with my brother." While she critiqued how those family care tasks and responsibilities fell to her, she also remembered finding a great deal of meaning in them, which was a theme running through the stories of women in different age cohorts and contexts, who told stories of being summoned to care *across their lives*, including in their households, paid work, and communities. Carrie's attention both to the conditions constraining her choices and to the ways she herself actively made meaning, is something we'll further explore in this chapter.

Carrie's story spoke clearly to how one's formative life history and social/material circumstances can shape how one comes to understand care or inhabit the role. For her, caring was central to who she was. She described how babysitting – or building her "babysitting empire" as she called it – had offered a way to launch herself on the path to redeem herself as a "responsible," "industrious" caregiver who could "get her own money," in relation to parents who weren't responsible, "never had money," and hadn't been able to meet her care needs. Laughing as she spoke, Carrie said, "'Cause at twelve, I've always been very industrious. You know, babysitters club! Here's my business model, you know, it worked for me." She also remembered that with "that first twenty bucks [she] made, [she] bought groceries for the family." Babysitting can be easy money, acquired because – without public or collective options – people need someone to care and pay girls cheap rates to do it.

It stood out in Carrie's story that caring was a way to distinguish herself from her parents or become "somebody." As an Indigenous woman, care work offered a clear path out of hardship – a way to alleviate disempowerment, materially sustain herself, and put herself on a path to social status or security in the face of social or economic conditions threatening her family's survival. She said she had felt like the "fairy godmother" as a caregiver. She had been good at responding to others and did so with ease. Care was a life path central to who she was, something she had staked her life on. That babysitting job meant something.

Yet when I spoke to Vicki, an AIDS activist in her sixties, she could hardly be bothered to talk about babysitting or any other care-related experiences. She had technically qualified for the study, and had an experience "stepping back" from social movement work when it was time for her to retire, but the word "care" didn't evoke much. When we first started speaking, Vicki said, "So, I started to think about [your topic of life stories of care] and I was like, 'Caring and being cared for? … No.' That doesn't really register with my life history." As she said, "I don't have a lot of specific memories around caring from my family life." I probed a bit more about her upbringing or how she might define the term. I also perked up in my seat when she mentioned she was the oldest daughter with three younger siblings. *Bingo*, I thought. *Babysitting*. "Okay!" I said, as if breathing a sigh of relief. "Did you babysit them or look after them?" Vicki paused. "Uh, *yeah*, I did?" she said. "I know I did but I don't have strong feelings or memories about it." This stumped me a bit at the time. It also raises questions about the very different ways women come to inhabit and interpret caring roles, *or not*.

With that, my goals in this chapter are to tease out differences in women's concerns and in their coercions into care work, as a way to foster solidarity amongst women and build awareness of how conditions matter. From the title of this chapter to the transdisciplinary modes of working in it, I am inspired by Sally Chivers (2023), who testifies to the importance of thinking "differently and more deeply about care stories" (221). Of particular note, Chivers speaks to the importance of developing and telling relational stories of care that are "about the relationship between care worker and cared for (sometimes the employer) as well as about how that relationship develops within a broader social and especially economic system" (222). Taking a relational approach, as Chivers notes, involves accounting "not only for relationships among people but also physical, social, political, and cultural conditions" (221).

Recognizing that there's no universal story when it comes to care, and aiming to think "differently and more deeply," I ask: How do women come to express different meanings of "care" or to inhabit caring roles in different ways? What do women's stories reveal about how gendered power relations operate? I will start by providing an overview of some of the individualizing tropes about "types" of women that circulated in the research I conducted. From there, I will reflect on how context matters in shaping how women are "summoned" into care, how they make meanings, and how they "inhabit" caring roles. My analysis in this chapter shines further light on structural and symbolic relations, and on intimate and institutionalized ones, that shape cultural assumptions around what makes a good/moral woman or what it means to care.

With these focal points, this chapter contributes to feminist scholarship that tracks shifting gender practices, meanings, and expectations as they change over time and vary across contexts (Bryant and Schofield 2007; Connell 2005). I draw particular inspiration from research that considers how gendered practices (including women's expressions of femininity) shift over time, with different gendered expectations at play. As a range of research illustrates, femininities are not "fixed" states of being but are "in tension," and those "tensions are important sources of change" (Connell 2000, 13). In speaking of differences in gender practices between generational cohorts, Connell (2005) notes that "there is contradiction, distancing, negotiation, and sometimes rejection of old patterns, which allows new historical possibilities to emerge" (24).

Gender practices – including the practices of caring or telling stories of care – are socially and historically mediated. Women's practices are defined and shaped differently in different contexts. As Angela McRobbie (1993) notes, "gender practices and meaning structures" change over time, with different narratives circulating among particular age-cohorts that reflect and shape different political, economic, and social periods. New emergent "modes of femininity," as they are put in practice, "tell us something of real significance about the society in which we now live" (McRobbie 1993, 156). For instance, some note that more recent modes of feminine expression combine masculine and feminine qualities to cultivate empowered feminine neoliberal subjectivities (Ringrose and Walkerdine 2008; Rivers-Moore 2010), which will also be apparent in some of the stories I present in this chapter.

In comparing the stories of women in different age cohorts, Jacqueline Kennelly (2014) illustrates how young women activists "continue to be tied to the gendered expectations that they care for others" (246–7), which she refers to as the "retraditionalisation of gender under neoliberal modernity" (248). She notes that, as care has shifted "away from the state and towards individuals," "women have come to play a central role" (246). Relatedly, Marjorie Silverman and colleagues (2020) show how "gendered expectations within a capitalist system" still play out for young adult carers, even with "feminist theorising and activism regarding the denaturalisation of care as women's work" (12). Their research shows how young women adhere to gendered expectations in ways similar to those in previous age cohorts. Drawing inspiration from these two studies, I consider in this chapter how different gendered meanings and expectations inform the practices of women in different age cohorts and contexts.

Women can be thought of as "summoned" to care, which is a term that accounts for the ways women are coerced, conditioned, or recruited to care for others, as well as the ways that they actively participate in the process (Tavory 2016; Winfield 2022c). Summoning gets at how the self (or a particular presentation of self) is evoked, as well as at how women inject new meanings into their experiences. Those who are summoned are themselves active in the process (Tavory 2016) when they make new meanings or refashion their roles. It's also notable that summonings happen intersituationally (Tavory 2016) or across contexts. Women aren't just recruited once and for all by a job advertisement; they are summoned across their lives in relation to other individuals, social institutions, structuring relations, and imaginaries. In the analysis that follows, I look both at how women are summoned to care and at how they inhabit those roles.

The word "inhabiting" calls to mind embodied practices of dwelling, living, or residing (Klostermann and Funk 2022). It's a term that can help account for the different ways people take on or relate to caring roles, whether with one foot out the door or with care as an all-encompassing life project. In terms of how people are drawn to inhabit particular feminized subject positions, not everyone has the same options, avenues, or possibilities available to them. As Alexis Shotwell (2013) writes, "the way one is gendered, or the gender expression one can produce, is in some real way shaped by the social location one occupies" (121). Embodied differences, including race, class, and gender differences, shape how one can present or position oneself, as well as how one is viewed by others.

"Some People Like a Big Frenzy" and Other Tropes

If a goal in this chapter is to counter individualizing tropes by telling more deeply contextualized stories of care and of how conditions matter, it's helpful to first consider the tropes and the ways women can be pitted against each other.

When I first started conducting this research, a long-time feminist sociologist suggested that my focus on the limits of care might help me to show that it's a type of person – an oldest daughter, with an alcoholic dad, passive mom, and early experiences of childhood neglect – who is susceptible to burning out. Even with her PhD in sociology and ten years of work in academia, she located the problem with the care sector in the flaws, deficiencies, or developmental wounds of women like me.

A long-time union researcher did the same. When I told her about my experience at L'Arche, she argued that someone like me, who went to university, should have had the wherewithal or class resources to navigate the care sector – to set boundaries or resign from the work before I burned out and became resentful towards the people I supported. "You shouldn't have let it get to that," she said, putting the onus on me as an individual. Drawing some distance, she seemed to suggest that suffering to the extent that I had shouldn't happen to the average person. She suggested that mine was a unique case, that there had to be something about me as a type of person that was the problem. She seemed to uphold the idea that "bad things don't happen to good girls" (Lopesi 2021, 113), similar to that Former Nurse and that Feminist Icon. I have to wonder if it perhaps comforted her to think that she herself would be smart enough to say no or set limits or figure out a way to keep herself safe. Perhaps there was comfort in her thinking my story was a story about a special kind of fucked-up person – not a story about institutionalized conditions that others might also be subject to.

I must admit though, I too sometimes felt like that wrong "type" of person when conducting this research. I questioned what was wrong with me or what I had done wrong that had led me to suffer to the extent I had. I blamed myself for burning out. I regretted that I went in hungry and looking for something that I didn't do more to keep myself safe, set boundaries, or say no. At the group home, offering to support that resident in the ICU had meant working fewer hours for less pay for a few weeks straight. After my interview at L'Arche, as I walked across the grounds with one of the L'Arche elite, I commented to him that L'Arche seemed like a campus, a real training ground for spiritual development. "A campus! What a *delightful* word choice," he had said. "It *is* like a campus," he offered, promising the world. I couldn't help but wonder if I'd missed some red flags or if a woman with more self-respect wouldn't have settled for that twin bed to begin with. *Six-foot-three with my feet hanging off? What was I thinking?*

I thought back to after my volunteer service year in LA. I dovetailed into that job at the group home, while other volunteers used their year of service to get a leg up on applications for law school, med school, or master of social work programs at top-tier, elite US universities. Those from elite families got out quick. I had to wonder if their parents had tipped them off that there was nothing there for them, that care work was a project with diminishing returns. I couldn't help but feel resentful that my working-class parents hadn't pointed me in the direction of a better life. I also felt sick thinking of how much I had inadvertently followed in the footsteps of my mom and grandma. When I first started in social justice work, I can remember thinking I was taking a counter path – that you wouldn't find me lording over a kitchen in lieu of expressing myself outside the home. It stung to think that the traps we fell into were different, but that – unlike my mom and grandma – I didn't even have a child of my own to show for all the work.

These were some of the individualizing understandings I was working against at the time of conducting my research. They were the subtext in my conversations with participants.

At the beginning of our second conversation, by way of hello, Gracie mentioned that she had just come from snuggling an "absolutely gorgeous, content, well-loved baby." From there, she said, "I talked to my friend Gina [who I, Janna, had also interviewed], and she was telling me what you guys talked about." *Boom.* It was a simple sentence, but it hit me like a punch in the gut. *Uh oh – where is she going with this?* I thought. I felt sick thinking of how I had played the "good girl" with Gracie (giving her space to frame her narrative and positioning myself as equally meek and well-meaning in response), but with Gina, we had been letting it rip, as we both expressed our resentment and bitterness, ranting and venting from line to line. "I just think it's *interesting* sort of where people's sense of commitment comes from," Gracie said. The word *interesting* landed like another punch. Speaking of caring for her mother, Gracie said, "It was an obligation, and *sure*, that's true. *To a point.* But, *for me*, when I was doing any of the things I was doing, it was always from a place of love. The obligation part never really came to mind for me. So same deal, you know, all the caring, you have to be self-less ... But just totally different feelings about it. Like I felt satisfied and content and rewarded for what I was doing. It made me happy, right?"

Gracie distinguished her own loving approach to caring for others from mine and Gina's. *Loving. Caring. Selfless. Rewarded. Happy.* From one word to the next, she cast herself as a moral, caring subject, and I felt more and more inadequate as she spoke – the wrong type of woman. I felt as though Gracie was scrutinizing and disciplining me for stepping out of line with my area of research and for failing as a caregiver. Her comments felt like critiques of my own work and life, of how I hadn't quite managed to pull off the moral, feminine ideals to which I had aspired. As I listened to her, I felt like I was being kicked out of the club after having tried so hard to live my life in a moral way – to be that *good*, that *moral*, that *remarkable*. And part of me wanted back in the club.

In response to Gracie, and as a way to show that I was moral and well-meaning too, I said, "Aw, you used the term 'soothing souls' where you were really connecting in a meaningful way. It wasn't just, 'all right, what's the job that needs to be done here?' Just a different quality to it." It was my way of trying to redeem myself by showing that I was moral enough to notice and value her moral approach. I also thought to myself after the conversation, *Really, Janna, still? You couldn't just let her comment about how caring she was hang there without countering that you had been caring too?* But I just couldn't. To me, this example speaks to more extended gendered power relations at play. It speaks to my own internalized views and my own ongoing investment in a particular narrative of myself as a caring and moral person. I too had been jostling for moral position. I too wanted to be good. And, although Gracie said it was the "same deal," which was a statement about conditions, I will reflect more below on the very different ways we were positioned – with different circumstances and ways of inhabiting the role.

I'll also admit that I felt a bit inadequate or like that wrong type of woman in conversation with Marilyn. "Knew it already" was how Marilyn, a retired nurse and former family caregiver around age seventy, talked about providing late-life family care. She spoke on a particular material basis, when we met at her beautiful condo building. I had passed the security gate and concierge desk on the way in, and had asked her about the walking track, swimming pool, and other amenities. She emphasized that she knew how to navigate the care sector, set boundaries, be smart, access resources, prepare for the caregiving work and the emotional process, and cope when the time came. *Nothing* surprised her. As she told it, there was *nothing* that she hadn't anticipated in caring for her parents. *Nothing.*

Much like my conversation with Gracie, I interpreted Marilyn's story as a critical commentary on my own failings as a care worker. It didn't occur to me at the time that her story – like my own and others – was a narrative production, not the reality. To Marilyn, I said, "Even as you've been talking about your approach to care, I've kind of thought, 'Oh, there is maybe a part of me that isn't as bounded or was kind of looking for something [to fulfil me] in the people I supported, or just maybe not as healthy boundaries.'" I positioned myself as a certain type of dysfunctional woman, and she didn't bail me out. Instead, letting me eat my words, she just said, "Some people like a big frenzy." Her story was a story about a type of person who flourishes, with me cast as the type who likes a big frenzy. We didn't say nearly enough about the very different conditions under which we were summoned to care, or about all the resources she had to pull things off.

I also felt a bit inadequate, albeit in a different way, in conversation with Julie, a former L'Arche assistant who was in her late twenties at the time of speaking to me. I blurted out my response to Julie's story without taking a breath: "Oh, *wow*, yeah, you certainly have me thinking about the toll that it takes on the body, or how exhausted you are the year afterwards or how it's not sustainable, so then you end up having to pay the cost, whether it's paying out of pocket for dental work or – and not even [having] the option to call in sick had you needed a mental health day or something." I know that I came on strong. The truth is, I was excited to speak to her, as we had both lived and worked at L'Arche, although in different communities. I cheered at some of the ways she put it, such as when she mentioned that she wanted more "reciprocity" in care, before giving the example of "even just being asked how [her] day was." We both laughed that it was something as simple as that, something as simple as having someone in the vicinity that might be able to ask how she was doing. I have to say, though, that I felt a bit caught off guard, or perhaps just ill-equipped for life in general, as our conversation progressed. Projecting onto her, and struggling to see past my own pain, I couldn't help but interpret her remarks as a commentary on who I was as a person or how I had navigated my work as a caregiver.

"I noticed red flags that were very disenchanting," Julie said, "I knew it wasn't going to be a comfortable place for a long-term commitment – knew it wasn't my version of community." As she put it, "the expectations of the community didn't really align with what I wanted to give. I was ready to give a lot of time and energy, but the expectations of what that meant didn't really line up with what the community wanted me to give." Julie emphasized that she was young. It was a learning experience. It was her first job after university. She was only twenty-two when she worked at L'Arche and "value[s her] own health and wellness differently now than [she] did before, when [she was] more susceptible to guilt trips." As Julie spoke, I just kept clocking things I had done wrong or hadn't thought to do. I hadn't noticed the red flags. I hadn't thought about how the community's expectations were different from mine. I hadn't been young and only twenty-two. Hers was an empowered story that I didn't know how to tell. And, much like my conversations with Gracie and Marilyn, we didn't reflect enough on the different life-spanning conditions of our lives, or the very different ways we were positioned in relation to care.

Sure, the conditions of our labour were similar as live-in assistants, but there were important differences in what care evoked for us or how we had been "set up" and summoned into the work. I had entered care work indefinitely and as a vocation, while Julie had moved into L'Arche for a one-year service year and with a set end date to her year-long contract. What care had represented to us, and the expectations that we had about what it would offer us, were vastly different. There was a piece there about the life-spanning conditions of our lives. There was something under the surface about the different ways we had been summoned to care and the different ways we had inhabited the role that invited further investigation. I had to ask: How is it that "care" evokes different meanings? How do conditions matter?

"Set Up" and Summoned across the Life-Course: Shifting Gender Relations and What "Care" Evokes

By comparing how women in different age cohorts (and different institutional contexts of care work) come to interpret and inhabit their work, further insight into care's shifting gendered organization emerges. In what follows, we'll start by looking at women's stories of being coerced to care, before considering differences in how these stories evoke meanings of care and in how women described inhabiting caring roles in particular institutionalized contexts.

"What's Not to Love?": Finding Meaning in the Care One Is Coerced to Provide

Something that stood out to me was that, even as the women in this study at times critiqued the broader structural patterns and gendered divisions of labour by which care tasks fell to them, they also often expressed finding a great deal of meaning in the care they were coerced to provide. This was the case for women in different age cohorts and contexts, who had been summoned to care in their households, in their paid work, and in their communities.

Most women in this study talked about growing up in households where housework and care were the domain of women, with men engaged in paid work and only (occasionally) "helping out" when they got home from work. As Marilyn said, "So I'd come home from high school and start the vegetables ... My dad said it was only fair to mother if we should do a little bit to start to help." In their early years, Troy recalled being "handed" babies when their dad lost his job and their mom opened a home day care. They mentioned that they didn't have a choice, as their mom just said, "No, you're looking after the kids when I can't do it." They also remembered that "there was a lot of pride" in the work, saying, "I think there probably was some like, 'Oh! I'm responsible enough that my mom needs me to come home and take care of kids.'" As they put it, "I think it added a lot of meaning to my life, a lot of responsibility, and kind of gave me a distraction from the not-so-great things in my life."

Pointing to the household care that daughters do, Gina shared that she had spent her childhood caring for "sick, sick, sick" family members and raising her baby sister, which she was often pulled out of school to do. She said, "When my sister was born, my mom handed her to me and said, 'here you go,' and that meant 'she's yours.'" As Gina said, "During the day, it was on me [to care for her], before my dad could get home and help out." Similar to Marilyn above, she noted how care work was her mom's responsibility, with her dad "helping out." Speaking in a critical tone, or as if to say "get this," Gina said, "And, because Mom was brought up this way, the boys didn't have to do anything, because you had to support your man." Yet, even with a critical edge to her comments, Gina expressed finding meaning in the support she provided. As she put it, "She was the baby, so what's not to love?"

Women in this study also emphasized finding meaning in paid care work that they entered into with limited other options. In speaking of her job at the group home, which was the only job she could find after university, Nora said, "I had so many friends out of university that couldn't get jobs in [town] that had to move away or were working minimum wage jobs, like serving or whatever." While Nora expressed having very limited employment options, she also remembered feeling like she had hit the "jackpot" in a small city where she and her friends had gone to university. She also said she had enjoyed "reimagining the role or kind of taking initiative and going above and beyond." Even in poking fun at the different gendered expectations at play within the work (such as in mentioning how a guy she had worked with – who didn't do as much of the emotional labour – had thought the job was a "breeze"), she expressed finding those aspects of the work meaningful. She remembered thinking, "I found my purpose; I found something I'm really good at that's really meaningful."

To give another example of someone finding meaning in paid care work, Marilyn, who was born in the 1940s, talked about entering into nursing, which she noted was one of the few paths available to women at the time. She said, "When I was maybe five, I told my mother I would be a nurse or an airline stewardess and she said, 'I think a nurse, dear.'" At that particular historical moment, women could be nurses, secretaries, or teachers. Those were the options. Yet, while Marilyn emphasized her limited choices, she too expressed finding meaning in the work and in her professional capacities. As Marilyn put it, "I certainly was given a lot of respect for my role that I played."

Those who talked about providing late-life care also framed themselves as finding meaning in the care they were obligated to provide. While Gracie acknowledged that she didn't have a choice and had to care and be selfless, she framed that as a preference and said that she would have done it "*just because* of the relationship" that she had with her mom.

Rhonda, who was in her late seventies at the time of speaking, also expressed finding meaning in the late-life care she provided to her late husband following his stroke. "I taught him how to work the wheelchair and use his foot to get around," Rhonda said. Even as she described a constant battle to discipline paid care workers – instructing them on how to appropriately bathe, toilet, feed, transfer, or care for her husband – she seemed to find meaning in having known the "right" way to care for him. "I'm giving you information that works. Use it," she had said to them. While Rhonda spoke in a somewhat crass register, my conversation with her jogged my memory of how meaningful some of those intimate tasks had been. She talked about finding a strategy to transfer her husband in and out of his wheelchair that worked better for him and for his body than the strategies the home care workers used. She was proud of knowing him so well and seemed to derive a sense of meaning and purpose from the support she provided.

With that, there is no question that the women in this study at times felt pressured or coerced to care with limited options *not* to care (whether in households, paid work, or their communities). Their stories reveal dominant gender norms, as well as inadequate public-sector supports for care that over-rely on the unpaid or underpaid work of individual women, and frame care as an individual, private responsibility.

Faced with urgent calls and coercions to respond to others' needs, these women were summoned to care in different contexts across their lives. Summoning was an active process, as they themselves made something of their experiences, loading them up with meaning, and playing an active role. Even those who were more critical or resentful of their coercions into care or of some aspects of their care expressed finding meaning in it. This insight connects well to Clare Stacey's (2005) finding that home care "workers have a conflicted, often contradictory, relationship to their work" (832). Further, as we will explore below, when it comes to making meaning of care work, women did so in different ways, and with different conceptual resources to draw on.

"Good Girls" and "Rebels": Recasting the Caring Role

It wasn't just that the women in this study expressed finding meaning in the care they had to provide; it stood out that they evoked very different, socially specific meanings in speaking of this care. The "carer as good girl" pattern was most evident in the stories of some women in the older cohort (born before 1964), while the "carer as rebel" pattern was evident in the stories of those in the younger cohort (born after 1982). I'm certainly not saying that all women of certain ages have the same ways of framing their lives, but their stories do speak to shifting cultural and political currents, and to how their formative life histories and social and material circumstances had shaped their imaginations for care.

Good girls. The "carer as a good girl" pattern was evident in the stories of most women in the older cohort, who presented themselves as emulating their mothers and spoke about the importance of family loyalty and bonding. Positioning herself as following in her mother's footsteps, Gracie remarked, "My mom was always taking care of somebody ... So, I have always been somebody who has wanted to take care of people." With the "So, I," Gracie framed caring as a natural inclination; she said that her mom "passed it on," that it was "just normal" for her, and "just became a part of" her. She also stated that she grew up "seeing, knowing, and believing that human beings were supposed to help to take care of the people that they love that needed help." In Gracie's story, family was conceived as the most important area of her life. To be positioned as the "good" caregiver in her family seemed to be a valued, desirable position, with cultural or moral accolades accompanying it.

Sheila also talked about emulating her mother and about caring out of loyalty and bonding. Speaking with affection for her mother, Sheila said, "I can remember other school kids walking [to and from school] with us, because they liked [my mom] so much. And there was one fellow who was the real bad boy of the school who always walked with her. He *loved* my mom." She framed the position of mother as an honourable, esteemed position – evoking images of her own good mother and sharing about her own practices as a mother. Much like Gracie, Sheila also expressed that she had always "been the caregiver." "I'm the one, you know, who brought home all the stray cats and looked after dolls and all that. I've been the caregiver since I was that high," Sheila said, pointing to her waist. Such a maternal discourse was supported by an ideology of family responsibility, as well as by a particular gendered division of labour that sees women shouldering responsibility for care. Good girls care.

Rebels. Speaking from different vantage points and with different points of emphasis, those in their late twenties and thirties (in the younger cohort) framed their recent paid work experiences in an alternative way. The term "rebel" captures the position that was constructed for them, and that they themselves co-constructed, in the precarious paid care work positions that they had entered in the late 2000s and early 2010s. In their stories, university served as a "framing institution" (Watkins-Hayes 2019, 151), giving them access to a lexicon that helped them to conceive caring as political work centred on listening and learning from society's most vulnerable. They drew on circulating narratives framing care as an anti-oppressive political practice, with paid care work offering a way to live out academic teachings on social justice, disability, power, and privilege.

It caught my attention that younger participants distinguished their approaches from conventionally feminine, maternal approaches to care, framing caring for others as an emancipatory political project. In speaking of caring for others across their life, Troy distinguished their caring approach from their mother's maternal, subordinate one that had centred on caring for family members or caring in apolitical volunteer roles. Troy recalled that their mom always volunteered and "put a lot of other people before herself." She was an elementary school supply teacher, ran a day care, and would volunteer at night with Girl Guides or at a local seniors' building. Troy poked fun at their mother's conviction that caring and having "other people come first" is "how you build community," which Troy didn't think was "completely healthy." For Troy, caring wasn't about a one-way flow of care as they met the needs of individual others, but about entering into more mutual relationships, and contributing to society through anti-oppressive political work. They talked about their "work with folks who are really not seen as people and are really devalued because they can't contribute to society in a capitalist way." Troy also underscored the importance of challenging racism, ableism, sanism, and classism, and of claiming solidarity with society's most vulnerable.

Others similarly framed care work as part of a political and intellectual project. For instance, Julie recalled that caring for others had been a way of resisting ableism and contributing to broader anti-oppressive work. She mentioned that she had been critical of dominant medical or behavioural-ist approaches to disability when she was in university, with readings that had said, "These are the symptoms, this is how you fix it, and this is how you create normal." She challenged dominant ableist understandings that framed disabled people as "problems" and that came with invitations to erase difference, manage behaviours, control others, or make them "quote-unquote normal." Similar to Troy, Julie had an understanding of oppression, privilege, and power. She cared as a way to rebel.

It's also worth reflecting on how one's formative life history and social/material circumstances shape (and at times undercut) the stories one tells. The "good girl" and the "rebel" – which are positions that seem to signify elite, white projects in the stories of some – aren't figures that everyone evoked in their stories or could easily inhabit.

Analysing Carrie's story helped me to think about this, as she shared about entering into a caring role in a context of material disadvantage and mistreatment. By putting those details on the record, she seemed to curb any reading of herself as someone creatively "refashioning" the role in the conventional ways introduced above. She went to university after entering into work as a care worker, and social justice discourses were less apparent in the stories she told about her foray into the work. Telling it like it is, and without overly intellectualizing it, Carrie said that after she moved in with her dad, her step-siblings, who lived with her mom, would often phone her to ask, "Can you drop off a roll of toilet paper? Mom's gone. We don't have this or that." She at times also framed caring for others as straight-up exploitation.

Gina did the same. In speaking of caring for her mother, Gina called attention to her limited material resources, limited options to share responsibility, and limited supports from others. She put in details that seemed to curb any reading of her finding it rewarding or being a (happy-go-lucky) "good girl." Instead, she described herself as "dumb enough to care for others." The part about how she could end up with a "fist in [her] face" from her ex-husband if supper wasn't on the table worked against some more conventional ways of reading her story. People need capital to buy into certain figures or to constitute themselves through the practices that make up such a figure (see Dosekun 2020). Good girls and rebels are two options, but you need the right material to weave those stories.

So, as we've explored, ideals of family responsibility ran through some accounts. Anti-oppressive ideals ran through others. It stood out that those in the younger cohort weren't constituting their femininity by being nice, passive, accommodating, or nurturing (Ringrose and Renold 2010). Nor were they evoking figures of the "truly feminine woman" or of one that "was childlike, nonassertive, helpless without a man, 'content in a world of bedroom and kitchen, sex, babies, and home'" (Bordo 2003, 170). In their stories, care was decoupled from maternal or conventionally feminine ideals. Their stories align well with the cultural sensibility of post-feminism, which declares women now free or empowered, and clears space for women to return to normatively feminine pursuits without compromising their empowerment (Dosekun 2020). On the surface, such stories of caring for others were not part of establishing a conventionally feminine self-image. They weren't stuck in the kitchens of their own homes or living out esteemed maternal projects.

That said, this is by no means an optimistic account of shifting dynamics or a kind of "progress" in the care economy. My argument isn't a hopeful one about the development of more "relational" or "mutual" forms of care, as we can see in these women's stories that the work of care *still* fell to them, with gendered divisions of labour. As some ways of orienting to care are contested, new ones emerge, creating different social relations, or even "traps," that shape and constrain women's lives.

The "Only One," the "Only Thing," or "Part of the Team":
Intimate and Institutional Relations

As we'll further explore, women's stories teach us about the intimate and institutionalized relations of their lives. In speaking of late-life family care roles, women often talked about being the "only ones," as they described feeling as though others were dependent on them for survival. Paid care workers in the younger cohort, on the other hand, tended to emphasize how care (as a vocation) was the "only thing" or only way of life. Expectations that one is the "only one" or that care is the "only thing" spoke to the nature of those care relationships, as well as to the institutionalized structures of care and cultural constructions of care shaping them. Such stories contrasted with ones in which women saw themselves as "part of the team," with options to share responsibility or lean on others while in that caring role.

Women's stories illustrate how expectations to care are contextually specific and "go both ways." By that I mean women face expectations to care in different ways and also have different expectations about what caring for others will offer them. As Martha McMahon (1995) writes, "men and women tend to experience themselves and self-other relationships in gendered ways because social situations are deeply gendered, both in the structures that organize them and in the expectations we bring to them" (269). Relatedly, Bev Skeggs (2004) writes, "Workers enter the labour market with different values ... making them more or less amenable to the potential for exploitation" (71).

It wasn't that those in paid care work roles didn't at times feel like the "only ones," or frame their work in that way. Troy, for instance, talked about a service user they supported, saying, "I had to help him do all his grocery shopping and all his appointments." As Troy said, "I kind of became his interpreter as well, because although he has dentures, people can't understand and then he gets frustrated with people, and I think he got very attached to me." Noting that they were the only one who could communicate with him and support him, Troy had serious concerns about "taking time off," as they felt "balls are going to get dropped" and "people aren't going to get the services they need." Other paid workers also expressed feeling irreplaceable in their roles. That said, what they most often spoke to, or what seemed to be most at stake or most holding them in their care work roles, was that care was a way of life, central to their identity. Care was the "only thing," as we'll look at below.

The "only one." Some but not all the family caregivers I interviewed remembered feeling integral and irreplaceable or like the "only ones" who could provide family care, with limited options to share responsibility. Gina indeed framed herself as the "only one" who could do it, in talking about caring to keep her mother alive. She said that she was forced to be the primary, full-time family carer after her mom had a stroke in the early 2010s, when Gina "sat there for days, telling her to breathe the right way." Gina's story was evidence of the state's over-reliance on unpaid family care, with care understood as an individual, private, family responsibility. Distinguishing herself from her siblings who couldn't do it, Gina said they were "crying and falling apart;" they couldn't "do Mom," couldn't "handle" her, so Gina did. She also remembered feeling like she had been left "stranded" by her siblings, "caregiving with *no* break." She was the "only one."

Gracie, who was in her mid-fifties at the time of speaking, also positioned herself as the "only one" in speaking of providing 24/7 care for her mother, with limited other supports and without the option to share responsibility. "She didn't have anybody else that could care for her," Gracie said. She also expressed that her mother's life was depending on her support: "I knew that I needed to be where I was, and I knew that her chances for rehab, survival, decent life really, really would be affected by my involvement or non-involvement, care or non-care." As Gracie said, "She would just call my name, right? She'd just be like, 'Gracie, Gracie,' and I would go running down the stairs."

Gina and Gracie both talked about keeping their mothers alive, with stories that had clear links to dominant ideals around family responsibility and to inadequate public-sector supports that over-rely on women to take responsibility for caring for their dependent family members "for free, on the basis of love and affection and reciprocity (Glenn 2010)" (Levitsky 2014, 7). Indeed, the state withdrawing responsibility for care (and downloading that responsibility onto individuals) is central to how such stories have taken shape. Pointing to policy shifts in Ontario, Marilyn emphasized that decades ago home care used to provide more supports (and hours of care per week) to families, with the state taking more responsibility. She noted that with the way those services have been clawed back, the onus now falls on women in the family to pick up the slack. Something as simple as the number of hours of public care offered to people who need it per day makes a difference in whether women are put in the morally fraught situation of having to "keep mom alive." We can also see how being positioned as the "only one" can make it hard for carers to set limits or to honour their own needs. The pressures are real.

As Gina said, "There's pressure from her, there's pressure from your siblings, if it's your mother. There's pressure from the outside to do right. And then the pressure on the inside and the physical and mental pressure you put on yourself to do the best … And in my case, it was my mother, so, you know, it wasn't like it was a job – a paid job – this was free, out of the goodness of my heart. And I had to, you know, you have to take all the crap that they're dishing." Gina mentioned the pressures she felt from all sides and the fact that family carers "have to take all the crap that they're dishing." Her comparison to paid care workers struck me, as some of the young paid care workers also framed themselves as having had limited options to step back, as we'll explore.

The "only thing." Taking what others are dishing and struggling to set limits were also clear themes in the stories of younger women who framed care as the "only thing" or central to who they were.

With care as the "only thing," Nora, who was in her mid-thirties at the time we spoke, remembered how care work came with a sense of self-worth, purpose, belonging, intimacy. It had been central to who she was as a person. "I never expected to find so much meaning and community," she said. She mentioned that she valued the relational aspects of the job, including "sitting with the people [she] supported, having a conversation, joking around, relating on a human, person-to-person

level." She said care work "felt like a privilege" and "felt really meaningful and really important." It was a way to contribute to disability justice and community-building, and she framed it as the most meaningful
and most energizing experience of her life. It was the first time in her life
she had ever experienced such a sense of purpose and meaning, and she
really felt like she was doing what she was born to do. Nora remarked
that it "turned into more of an identity or something that became a
really important part of [her]." As she said, "I felt more empowered
or more capable, or had something to say, had something to give, you
know, at least more than I've ever felt in my life." She framed it as a time
of personal growth and remembered learning "so much about [herself]
and about other people." Care became the "only thing."

For Nora and some others in the younger cohort, care was framed
as interwoven with one's sense of self. Caring wasn't just a job, and
wasn't just about meeting others' needs, but was a site of self-expression,
intimacy, and advocacy. It also stood out that, similar to others in the
younger cohort, Nora described feeling irreplaceable and integral to
others, with work bleeding into her non-work life. Care work was an
all-encompassing life project that extended beyond the clock:

> I think the organization didn't have really any sense of boundaries,
> because it was sort of constructed as this, like, a sense of community and
> family and we're all in this together and we're all supporting each other …
> A lot of people, their personal and professional lives like bled into each
> other a lot … I'd come home from work and I didn't always turn off, right?
> Like I'd spend a lot of the night worrying about, "Did I," you know? Did
> I checkmark all the meds? Did I do all this stuff? Forget to do something?
> Is so-and-so okay? It was just not trusting that things could go on okay …
> I think there was a lot of bleed-through.

Nora pointed to a range of unpaid work she did off the clock, as well
as to the lack of boundaries at the organization where she worked
that led to her taking an individual sense of responsibility and finding it hard to turn it off. In a threadbare sector, and at an organization
with low wages and conditions of overwork, Nora faced heightened
expectations to work for free or to "care for nothing" through unpaid or
additional work (see Baines 2004), and with the "costs and risks downloaded on [her as] the worker" (Baines et al. 2019, 885).

Troy also expressed feeling like care was the "only thing." They too
talked about finding a sense of purpose in care work, and about how it
was central to their sense of self. In speaking of the service users they
supported, Troy said, "I've learned more from them than I think they

ever learn from me." I of course related to their stories about care as a self-making project. "It did almost feel like this magical space with what was possible with relationships – this vulnerable, intimate, cool thing, you know?" I said to Troy. I too had felt like I was offering something that felt unique, like space had opened up or this was what I was meant to do. I also related to deriving a sense of worth, as I remembered thinking, "Wow, they see something in me, you know?" Troy and Nora both agreed with what a privilege it had been. I also think these stories raise questions about how care can be organized responsibly, given how transformative it can be.

Elsewhere, I have traced forms of boundless work organization in contemporary care organizations that call on employees to put in more time, engage in unpaid or additional work, identify with their roles, and take individual responsibility for the work and the risks (Klostermann and Funk 2024; Klostermann et al. 2025). Such conditions are apparent in the stories of younger workers. We can also see how care is "boundless" in that it deeply shapes one's sense of self and sense of future possibilities. Having care as the "only thing" can make women vulnerable.

Yet I also saw promising examples in which people talked about caring as "part of a team," without the same sense of stakes or challenges when it came to being able to set limits or step back.

"Part of a team." While those in the younger cohort talked about paid care work as a self-making project, those in the older cohort framed their past paid work experiences as well-bounded professional work. Rhonda and Marilyn, two retired nurses in their seventies, noted that they had worked their set hours, knew their place, and retired when it was time for their pensions. Neither framed the work as interwoven with their sense of self. Instead, they described teamwork as part of systems with built-in professional boundaries or ways to say no. Marilyn mentioned that "within a support system, [she] never felt overly threatened," and always had the option to say no. Rhonda said, "Cops and nurses are kind of the same kind of people; they get married all the time. It's a matter of fact … Firefighters too … Being a nurse, it's difficult to put the right hat on at the right time, right? And you're supposed to do as you're told by the doctors." Rhonda expressed a professionalized understanding of nursing as a form of employment and didn't once talk about expressing herself or following her life's purpose. Her sense of what the opportunity was about – doing as she was told – signals what she had expected in return, which was different from others who oriented to care as central to their sense of self. Rhonda had not only faced particular expectations to care, but also had particular expectations of what caring for others would bring.

As I read and re-read the transcript of my interview with Rhonda, I realized that I had been loading up care with specific meanings based on my own past care work experiences, in ways that were different from how she framed her experiences as just a job or as work she had done as part of a team. I asked Rhonda how she navigated "being in the presence of some who were really suffering or really in a lot of pain" and interjected with comments about how "other-oriented" relationships can be "energizing or nourishing." Those were my words, not hers. I was the one orienting to care as a self-making project and loading up care with certain intellectualized or moralized meanings. Rhonda's own ways of talking about nursing as paid and professional work were different, with different intimate and institutionalized structures shaping how care played out in that role.

"Patient contact" is how Rhonda talked about her ties with the people she supported. Speaking with a sense of ownership or power, Rhonda stuttered and mocked a patient, saying, "Rhon- Rhon- can I have a hug, Rhon?" Raising her eyebrows, she said, "The hug was more for him than it was for me." The way she claimed power over others stood in contrast to those in the younger cohort who talked about cultivating mutual, reciprocal relationships across difference, or about being there to learn.

Seeing herself as "part of the team" in a different context, Marilyn said how caring for her parents had been a shared responsibility – divided up between her and her siblings. "It was teamwork all along," she said, "so, that helps with caregiving, doesn't it? When you've got that support?" When her parents lived in a private retirement home, the phone calls in the middle of the night had been few and far between. "There was staff there, so the initial issue had been addressed by staff before they called me."

The importance of being able to share responsibility for care also stands out when I think about my conversation with Sheila. While Sheila asked, "So sometimes I think, did I take *too* good care of her?" it stood out that she had cared for others on a particular material basis. She had mentioned welcoming her mother into her family home, building a state-of-the-art granny suite, hiring "the cleaning lady" (who she already had a great relationship with) to help out, and later moving her mother into a private, urban retirement residence only five minutes away from her home. Care, for her, was also a shared responsibility, with collective backing and supportive conditions to pull it off. It's no wonder she brushed off my questions about whether she was resentful!

So, some former nurses and some family caregivers talked about having no trouble setting boundaries or limits on the care they provided.

Others described caring in positions in which boundaries, independence, and distance from the people they supported were harder to sustain or nearly impossible to imagine. Expectations to simply "clock in" or share the load were quite different from expectations to "go in with [one's] whole self all the time" (as Troy put it) or to care for others as part of an intimate self-making project at an "organization without boundaries" (as Nora recalled). Keeping your mother alive is a different game too. In speaking of the importance of challenging social policies that assign individual responsibility, Sally Chivers (2021) writes, "The dominant emphasis throughout the pandemic was, as ever, on the role of families rather than on broader understandings of the way in which humans need to relate in order to thrive, well beyond the conjugal imaginary" (174). Just as she underscores the importance of exposing shortcomings in social policies that assign individual responsibility for caring to families, we can see in women's care stories the importance of challenging other ways of individualizing responsibility or narrowing women's options.

Not everyone was "set up" to care against all odds at the expense of themselves until reaching a point of depletion. Not everyone had super-sized expectations about how care would fulfil them. But some did. In some women's stories, caring was a "salient identification" (Winfield 2022c) or something with real stakes. It was hard for them to imagine alternatives (whether having someone else step in or heading in a different direction in life). It's also notable that some *paid and unpaid care workers alike and in different contexts* described situations that were hard to think outside of, whether as the "only one" or with care as the "only thing." These were incredibly vulnerable positions to be in that cry out for rethinking the social practices and cultural politics shaping care *across contexts*. They also show the need for fostering solidarity amongst women in different paid or unpaid caring roles and age cohorts.

Rethinking Individualizing Tropes, Imagining Conditions to Pull Things Off

With the goals of countering individualizing tropes, identifying grounds for solidarity, and examining multiplicities under the surface of women's stories, the analysis in this chapter has shone a light on how the ways women understand and inhabit caring roles are profoundly shaped by gendered power relations in particular contexts and at particular social and historical periods. We looked at some tropes, as well as at stories of women who found meaning in care they were coerced to provide. We also considered variations in women's experiences, as they were shaped by symbolic circulating narratives, and by the nature of intimate and institutionalized relations.

Of note, women in this study were at times actively countering individualizing tropes and telling stories about how context matters. I learned a lot from them on this front. Carrie mentioned that when she first started recovering after exiting care work, she had wondered if there was a "beacon on her head" or something she had done to invite being mistreated. She remembered that it was "humiliating," that she felt "dumb," and that a friend had said to her, "You're crazy. *Wow*. You're *fucked*." In the context of our conversation, I interpreted Carrie as actively naming and countering such individualizing tropes about "types" of women, smirking as she spoke. Putting those details on the record seemed to be a way of saying, "I felt dumb *at the time*, but know how goofy that sounds now," or "*she* thought I was crazy and fucked up, but I think you'd agree, Janna, how wrong she was." Our conversation created a different context for that narrative.

It meant a lot to be in conversation with her and with others who were challenging individualizing tropes, telling fuller stories, and expressing compassion for themselves. When Troy questioned if they cared for others because, for whatever reason, they didn't feel cared for, I couldn't help but relate. I also cheered at the fact that, as soon as Troy's question about not feeling cared for while growing up left their mouth, they interjected, laughing and joking that I was probably going to analyse their comment. "Oh my gosh," I roared, laughing. It was more than a story about the type of person they were with a distancing or pathologizing analysis from me to follow, as we both seemed to be working through the shame that was supposed to keep us quiet. "If feminism is about the reclamation and redefining of power" (Lopesi 2021, 46), it was feminist work we were doing together.

Through these research conversations, participants and I were also at times raising questions about what kind of conditions would support us. In a recent chapter led by Susan Braedley, we consider the need for structural and process conditions to make joy possible in long-term care, identifying belonging, purpose or meaning, sharing, and pleasure as central to joy (see Braedley et al. 2023). As we write, "To live, and not just exist, humans need purpose, meaning, connection, and pleasure," which is true for carers and people who rely on care (152). It's a perspective worth considering in the face of care staff being run off their feet, "too weary and overworked to experience meaning" (161) or to build relationships with others as part of their work.

That said, to build on some insights presented in chapter 4, some of the stories presented in this chapter raise questions about whether finding (moral) meaning in caring for others without other sources of meaning outside of care, and without adequate conditions or the option to share responsibility, can make carers vulnerable or make it hard to set limits. This was something that participants were often thinking through. "I don't know if there's a way for us to really completely protect ourselves from the impact [caring] has on our physical, mental, spiritual selves," Troy said. Nora made a similar point, when she questioned if "having too many boundaries takes away connection or is sort of a detriment to care work." It's worth asking how we can help women go into this work with their eyes open to it, or with the tools to reflect on the expectations they themselves bring. Rather than an unwavering promotion of joy, I question how care would be organized differently if the different ways women are "set up" and "summoned" were taken into account.

While Rhonda talked about "doing as you're told," Nora mentioned feeling "more empowered or more capable ... than [she had] ever felt in [her] life." My research suggests it makes a difference if someone knows whether something is a shit gig (and has modest expectations about what it will offer them), or whether they enter into a situation with high hopes about how the work will fulfil them. It's worth considering whether we need some fine print around the push for meaning-making, in light of how harmful care relationships can be without adequate conditions, supports, and resources. It's worth asking: What conditions are needed to support women in wearing our hearts on our sleeves or engaging in care as meaningful work that can be a site of transformation, creativity, learning, and joy? How might we ensure carers are adequately supported, in contexts where care can be a site of intimate self-making and relationality?

Final Thoughts

This chapter reflected on care relationships as women come to inhabit and interpret them, with the goal of telling fuller stories about how context matters. With a focus on how women evoke meanings of care and reflect on their coercions into care, this chapter illuminated how carers face and hold different expectations at different times. The care economy is by no means the same for everyone, as the positions co-constructed in it are different for women in different age cohorts and institutional contexts.

My analysis raises questions about when/whether talking about care as an ethic is worthwhile. Women are often interpreted as responding to a calling, as though making moral choices or "choosing" to work in fields that pay less. While "morality" implies a choice, it's clear that moral elements are always in conversation with structural constraints.

With that, this chapter showed the utility of developing more nuanced, context-specific stories of care. Such stories show the power of dominant circulating meanings, of formative life histories, and of local specificities. They also show how, to transform care, we need to develop a more refined language for understanding and talking about carers' unique situations, formative life histories, and expectations about what caring for others will involve. We need tough and tender conversations between paid *and* unpaid care workers in different age cohorts, as I will explore in the closing chapter, and as the "Care Junkie Recovery Group" reading guide in appendix 1 is designed to help facilitate.

Conclusion: A Counter-Politics Playbook?

This book started at the limits of care. I shared in my memoir that some of my lowest points as a care worker were passing all those burn-out tests, crying in a sloppy, out-of-control way in a Starbucks, and raging under the surface at dinner parties. I should maybe add that there was also the time that I ripped the carpet out of my bedroom at L'Arche. And when I say "ripped the carpet out," I don't mean it metaphorically. For months, it had bothered me that the disabled people we lived with and supported had new laminate flooring, while me and the other live-in helpers had crappy old carpeting that looked like it was from the seventies. Mine was a bright turquoise shag carpet that prickled to touch. I inquired a few times in team meetings about when they planned to replace it. I also started noticing how the guestroom across the hall from me had the loveliest wooden floorboards. There seemed to be so much potential under those carpets. Something rustic and retreat-like even. Like a character in Charlotte Perkins Gilman's story, "The Yellow Wallpaper," I ripped that baby out. Over the last ten years, I've often thought about that as a sign of just how much I had lost it and just how entitled I had become in an organization that had taken so much from me. There was something irresponsible about ripping it out, as I was putting my problems on others and having them clean up after me – not just in an abstract way, but with the carpet and foam pad tucked behind the shed in the backyard ready for someone else to pick up. That version of myself is a character that I can hardly recognize or locate now, but I have so much compassion for her.

In chapter 2, "Towards a Counter Politics of Care," I shared that my research project was motivated by my struggles both as a care worker and as an emerging care scholar. I also shared a story Carrie told about waking up on the floor of that Walmart. For both of us, care *still* had a hold long after we had resigned. There was something about *still* feeling hooked or stuck that demanded my attention, just as there was something about dominant, hegemonic (moral, feminine, privatized) understandings of care that seemed to invite a disruptive, counter-story-telling approach. This book has been my way to respond to those problems, sticking with things a little bit longer. My overarching goals were to reflect on care's inequitable gendered organization, identify and challenge dominant tropes, assumptions, or expectations around gendered care work, and open possibilities for more equitable, emancipatory futures.

To come full circle, I'll reflect in this chapter on key insights and implications – on what the research reveals and on the power of the process. I'll consider the "so what" and the "now what." I'll ask: What can we – collectively and individually – do with all this information, other than rage? Where does this take us?

What the Research Reveals

Taken together, the chapters in this book interrogated gendered power relations and their constraining effects on women's lives, life trajectories, and imaginations. We looked head-on at women's agency, as we inhabit, negotiate, and resist dominant structures and meanings of care. We also moved beyond a focus on direct care in practice or on everyday work/organizational conditions, to learn from women's stories of care across the life-course, while orienting to women as political actors engaged in a politics of responsibility. I used a feminist sociological approach to examine women's lives as a serious subject – revealing how women are pressured into staying in care roles, as well as how we interpret and come to talk about our experiences.

Insights from feminist political economy supported me in considering how conditions matter, with feminist rhetorical approaches helping me to analyse women's stories. My analysis shows the value of weaving approaches from the arts, humanities, and social sciences to link women's counter stories and care-negotiation strategies to social and material conditions in the care economy, as well as to dominant circulating narratives. Attending to care as work, *and* to shifting conceptions of care that are remade in context, proved generative. With a focus on gender as a social relation, we traced intimate and institutionalized relations, as well as symbolic and structural ones. Narrowing in on the constructedness of people's stories and on intimate self/other relationships was part of my contribution.

Rather than focusing on care providers in a particular job (e.g., personal support workers) or a particular care setting (e.g., group homes),

I considered women's stories of paid and unpaid care work across contexts and sectors and at different social and historical junctures. Juxtaposing the stories of women in a younger age cohort with women in an older age cohort helped to reveal shifts in Ontario's care economy and in cultural or political currents. Comparing the stories of unpaid family carers with those of paid staff illustrated how moral, gendered expectations can extend beyond particular roles or realms. It was striking that women in different paid and unpaid care roles, and in different contexts, at times described similar challenges with boundary setting or with sharing responsibilities for care; they also at times told stories that served similar social functions. Had I focused only on family carers, a simple solution might have been that paid workers need to step in (indeed, we need more investments in a paid, publicly funded workforce), but there were no easy answers here, as we can also see how context matters, and how seemingly similar contexts can be night and day for women who have been set up or summoned differently. In some contexts, but not all, it's easy for women to leave, with stories they can hardly be bothered to tell. In others, we heard about blocked exits or just how ugly things can get. Conditions really matter, and they profoundly shape the stories women tell or the possibilities or paths we can imagine. Stories hold invitations about how responsibilities are understood and assigned and about how life can be otherwise. We need conditions for more imaginative stories and more imaginative stories about conditions.

We can also see how eliciting, telling, and learning from counter stories can be generative. Throughout this book, I've engaged women's counter stories of reaching their limits, stepping back, or otherwise renegotiating responsibility for care across their lives. These stories challenge and rub up against normative caring ideals and assumptions. I worked to identify dominant conventions, such as when I learned from my own and others' knee-jerk reactions or from the occasional "flinch factor" response. I also told stories to challenge dominant understandings about women's endless, selfless caring or about the power dynamics at the heart of care. Along the way, I've taken aim at dominant relations and narratives that socialize women into providing care against all odds and without adequate supports or outlets outside of the work. I've challenged tropes about "heartbreakers leaving," about the "privilege" of exiting, and about the "types" of people who thrive and the "types" who fail.

My analysis of women's accounts of reaching their limits made visible narrative silences and moralizing tropes that teach us about care's social organization. Stories about the body saying no, about not being able to turn water into wine, and about having guilt on top of that are ones that stick with me – ones that speak to the need for dramatically improving care conditions and for stretching imaginaries of care to ensure women are supported in setting limits and in talking about their own needs and the fullness of their experiences.

With a focus on stepping back or loosening the ties that bind, I analysed how women put time and energy into renegotiating their own and others' care needs, reorienting to their moral sense of selves and self-expectations and rethinking moralized expectations to care. My analysis challenged an assumption in feminist care scholarship that leaving care is possible only for those with social status and privilege. I also illustrated how care is always contested, always negotiated. Care is a domain of struggle.

From there, with a focus on thinking "differently and more deeply about care stories" (Chivers 2023, 221), my goal was to present fuller stories of care, and of how conditions matter, as a way to foster solidarity among women in different age cohorts and with different care experiences. While some desire to care, or don't mind – as caring has its benefits – it is still inevitably wrapped up in coercion at the level of (moral, feminine) self-fashioning. We also saw how moral or gendered expectations are contextually specific and "go both ways," as women face expectations and have different expectations of what caring will offer them back.

My analysis speaks to the necessity of thinking across contexts of paid *and* unpaid care work, and of getting in the room with other women to swap stories, even if we occasionally wind up jostling for position or rubbing one another the wrong way. This project also speaks the necessity of developing a language for care that includes limits, boundaries, and consent. We need definitions of care work that are collective in the fullest sense of the word – that move beyond describing "recipients" of care or the tasks involved in caring, or even the sense of responsibility one feels in caring for others, to include other intersecting, structuring relations, *as well as limits and boundaries.* Care isn't truly caring unless carers are free to choose *not* to care. We can see the need for exits, off-ramps, limits, and boundaries, as other advocates and scholars recognize ("Charlottetown Declaration" 2001; see also Funk et al. 2024). "If you're going in alone, don't go" is a phrase that comes to mind when I hear of individual workers or family members being funnelled or wedged into self/other, individual care relationships of the "you're the only one who can do it" variety or "care is the only thing" variety. I would argue that such individual arrangements aren't actually "care" and that going "in" or taking on responsibility in that way isn't "caring." Such conditions are dangerous and unacceptable for both the provider and the receiver; they are also evidence of the failures of welfare states and our failure to imagine care in more equitable or even emancipatory ways. If relationality, interdependency, or consent were taken seriously, carers would have not only options to withdraw or suspend their care work without guilt or shame, but also other sources of worth and recognition. Being able to leave is an indicator of gender equity; conditions should be good enough to ensure women can leave or are free to go. We not only need institutional supports for carers in their work but need liveable story structures to ensure the flourishing of all involved.

We've also explored how care as a gendered ethic that operates in the social realm can and does negatively affect individual women's lives. In saying that, I acknowledge that the ethic of care framework makes a significant contribution in rethinking notions of what counts as moral or what counts as contributing to political life. It's an important moral and political philosophy, useful in its applications to democratic life and structural changes. The care ethic makes sense as a political philosophy, as care is socially necessary labour, and we need social policies and arrangements that ensure the democratic provision of care for those who need it. I also note that Joan Tronto's (1993, 2013) work is about *democratically* imposed responsibilities to care. It is care as a collective responsibility that she is promoting, and she doesn't use the word *coercion*. The care ethic works well as an orientation similar to how the ethic of justice was intended.

That said, my analysis raises questions about the experiential underpinnings of care as an ethic, given how care is constituted at the level of individual women's subjectivities. Women's stories speak to the grip of moral expectations for women to care, and they raise questions about whether "care as an ethic" should apply at the level of individual women's lives. What is notable here is that "moral injunctions, not to act unfairly toward others, and *not to turn away* from someone in need" (Gilligan 1982, 20, emphasis added) can be quite constraining, and even harmful, when lived out or pushed to the limit in wider conditions of social neglect or without options for carers to share responsibility. Moralized understandings of care need some fine print. And while some scholars may scoff that of course the ethic of care is a political philosophy, I note that not everyone has access to conceptual resources or narratives that would help with interpreting it that way. There is a real need for more expansive public conversations around care and leaving care.

While care relationships can be sites of creativity, co-learning, and social transformation, not to mention self-making, belonging, meaning-making, and joy, they are wrapped up in inequitable divisions of labour, status and wealth, and caught up with gender, culture, ethnic norms, and moral, political positions, with carers caught in the mess. We see these contradictions clearly in women's stories and care-negotiation strategies. It's all good to recognize or promote care relationships as sites of transformation, but in addition to this whole-hog promotion, it's worth asking how structures and meanings of care can be rethought in ways that stop setting women up for such intimate losses. *How can care be organized responsibly, given how transformative it can be?*

One clue is in women's stories that illustrate the need to promote gender equity in a much broader sense – not just on the clock or in care relationships, but over the course of women's lives. Beyond recognizing, valuing, or redistributing the work of care, this calls for countering and dismantling women's subordination, as it extends beyond any particular care work role or realm. As we've explored, women need other outlets and options for work, worth, meaning, purpose, and connection, as well as for self-expression or social standing. We need liveable lives, and how society structures our worth or non-worth beyond care and across our lives is part of the story.

Taken together, my research suggests that care work is socially necessary labour – central to maintaining people and populations – but its organization through gendered, moral, and material coercions must be undone. It also suggests that feminist researchers and advocates need new approaches to do so. The conceptual and methodological approach that I've developed and employed in this research is part of my contribution and something that I think has tremendous power for researchers, advocates, care workers, and others.

The Power of the Process: A Counter-Politics Playbook?

The research I presented in this book involved a range of strategies, from recognizing the power of stories, to staying present to the disruptively disorienting experiences of our lives, to orienting to people as storytellers and political actors engaged in a politics of responsibility. The project also involved reflecting on my own and others' shared implication in the social relations of our lives, telling fuller, more deeply contextualized stories, contextualizing and recontextualizing, opening to the unexpected, learning from my own and others' knee-jerk responses, and pointing to possibilities. These can be thought of as strategies in my "counter-politics playbook."[1]

---

1 I draw inspiration for this term from Susan Braedley and Tara McWhinney's (2023) analysis of neoliberal profitization strategies in Saskatchewan's long-term care sector, which they refer to as the "privatization playbook."

The strategies I employed were also ways of taking responsibility and being accountable to the relationships I was bringing about. There was no neutral, innocent position to occupy (Code 2006, 219) as I put my "subjectivity ... on the line" and assumed responsibility for the world I was helping to bring about (275). In this project, advancing and enacting a "counter politics of care" approach has been a way of taking responsibility. I've worked hard to try to be accountable and take responsibility in the "production, circulation, and acknowledgement of claims to know" (Code 2006, viii). That said, the project wasn't simply about taking responsibility or being responsive, accountable, or otherwise of service *to others*. Instead, my approach offered a way to show up more fully, as an embodied researcher, artist, and human. Karen Barad (2007) writes that questions of responsibility and accountability are "not about representations of an independent reality but about the real consequences, interventions, *creative possibilities*, and responsibilities of intra-acting within and as part of the world" (37, emphasis added). I think her point about "creative possibilities" is an important one. Through creative critical work, this research has involved "bringing new stories, relationships, and worlds into being" (Doucet 2018, 749–50). As I've come to appreciate, taking responsibility centrally involves ushering in and opening to creative possibilities. The work of critique can be part of this.

Another important strategy in my "counter-politics playbook" was telling fuller, more nuanced and situated stories of my own and others' lives. In a podcast episode about creativity, self-discovery, and reinvention, Zoe Lister-Jones talks about how resonance is in the specificity; it is the specificity of our stories that creates the universal connection, not the other way around (Roll 2023). As this project has progressed, I've worked to write more honestly and specifically, with the stories in this book undergoing multiple, multiple revisions.

Sharpening the singularity of our stories, and telling fuller ones, is central to enacting a counter politics of care. For me, this process has also involved rethinking my relationship to my sense of self and to the reader. As I was writing this book, I drew inspiration from a journal article written by Talia Schaffer (2019) entitled, "Why Lucy Doesn't Care: Migration and Emotional Labour in *Villette*." In the article, Schaffer writes, "But the story of *Villette* is, in part, the story of Lucy gradually managing to imagine a different type of reader. It becomes possible for her to narrate her story because she comes to believe in a reader who is like a lover, not like an employer" (86). This observation resonated with me, as I also noted a shift in conducting this research from my feeling alone in my experience towards recognizing and seeking out commonalities with others and trusting the reader with more vulnerable or tender parts of my story. The suggestion that got me was from two anonymous reviewers, who recommended that instead of presenting my memoir at the end of the book, I should put that material first to help readers understand how I came to the topic. This felt like a major shift, as it meant trusting the reader with a tender part of my story to start, rather than waiting until the end to mention just how much the experience had meant, and just how painful it had been. This changed things. It really did. I wouldn't have been able to write that version a few years ago, but it changed things to introduce a vulnerable young Janna to start.

I must admit – earlier versions of my memoir material read more like victim impact statements, with accounts of care broadly defined but without as many specifics about how I had inhabited particular roles and relationships. For several years after resigning, it was too painful for me to write about the honeymoon stage or admit just how transformative the experience had been initially, given how poorly it had turned out. It was my friend and colleague Saro who encouraged me to add more of my personal context to the study, to write about my spiritual connection to care work – about what drove me and what I desired. When I did, I was struck by what a dedicated kid I was, how idealistic and open to the world I'd been. There had been a fire in my belly, as I had wanted to give my utmost somewhere. I noticed that my story was a story about femininity, whiteness, class, and age – about a young white woman in her twenties who was trying to figure out who she was and how to live. It changed things to take Saro's advice and the advice of those reviewers who had shown care for me and my story.

Writing about the tender-to-the-touch parts – about my light-hearted, idealistic formative years – also created space for me to write more fully about the counterpoint to that. To put in the part about Shelly. When I first read that part aloud to myself, I choked up, thinking about how much I've been through.

I also remember tearing up when I came across an article about spiritual abuse that talked about how it involves the distortion of spiritual authority to manipulate and control others (Barnett 2023). I hadn't thought of myself as abused in that way as a care worker, at least not until I got to the part in the article about how some who have experienced spiritual harm can find it helpful to "put the spiritual language aside for a season" or "set down some of these former practices that have deeply shaped you" (Clinton Chen as cited by Barnett 2023). I had to admit how much I had set down, how many practices and parts of myself had gone into hiding.

Along the way, I've also had to admit that I haven't just been getting it handed to me but have actively been working to resist dominant power structures and narrative frameworks, as defined by those in power. At the risk of a future reader commenting that I should have been too smart to have suffered – that there must be something uniquely wrong with me – I added in more details about my art-making and advocacy work. I put in the scene in which I staked my claim as an artist in conversation with Martha. I admitted to the reader and to myself how much art and writing had been (and still are) driving my life. Putting those parts in not only helped me to reflect on my own agency, individuality, and power, but also came with an ethical demand to call attention to women's agency, individuality, and power in telling their stories.

With each version of the book I've tinkered with, I've added more about my friends and mentors who have helped me in framing and situating my experience. I can't help but picture my friend Taylor who wrote me to say, "go harder and be more dramatic," and my friend Catherine who once messaged me to say, "stay mad and say more and never stop." The ways I've been supported are part of the story.

Like a stand-up comic learning from the laugh of the crowd, I've put myself out there, made offers, and learned from my own and others' knee-jerk responses. There was pleasure in "learning as I went along, asking the hard questions, not knowing what was coming next" (Lorde 2012, 98). This was the case in the "flinch-worthy" performance, in the conversations that I had with other women, and in the however many encounters along the way. Putting ourselves out there, and putting the emphasis somewhere, offers a way of working things out, refashioning ourselves, our relationships, and our understandings. It's in conversation with others that we can learn new insights about our lives, and about how things are organized.

There was something about listening to, transcribing, reading, and re-reading my conversations with others that helped me to see myself more clearly. Reviewing line after line, I couldn't help but notice the way I said "yeah, yeah" to agree with others, or the way I at times started off a sentence by making a run for it, talking about honouring my own needs or desires, and *then*, as if not wanting to get accused of being selfish or privileged or emotionally reckless, wrapped up the story by speaking of my commitment to other-oriented work or to the more pressing needs of those who deserve to have their care needs met. I couldn't simply talk about exiting or about my own needs, without noting that the people I supported had real needs too. "I mean, you want to affirm your own desires and honour your own ideal vision for your life," I said to Nora, "but you still have this understanding of how some people are more devalued than others, you know, this real responsibility to be in relationship with others, you know?"

What stands out is the power of having interviewed women – ages twenty-seven to seventy-eight – who reflected on paid *and* unpaid care work *across their lives*. Being part of those tough and tender conversations helped me to notice more common ground not just with those who share my sensibility or came of age around the same time, but with others who had crafted their lives in different ways. Betty. Rhonda. Marilyn. Sheila. Judy. Gracie. Gina. Vicki. Carrie. Nora. Troy. Julie. I also think of my sister, Claire, my mom, Kathy, and my grandmas, Irene and Gail. As I think of past conversations, and ones to come, I'm convinced that telling the stories that are ours to tell, and attending to commonalities and differences, can help us to transform our sense of selves, our understandings, our relationships. Such conversations help to create the conditions needed to build solidarity across fault lines – putting contradictions on the table, while putting our lives in common.

Moving forward, I can see the value in weaving approaches from the arts, humanities, and social sciences to rethink the stories we tell about care and to tell new ones or fuller, more imaginative ones. I can also see how much there is to learn from those positioned differently in the care economy, including those loosely understood as needing care, shouldering or shirking the work of care, or resisting and revising care responsibilities. Further research is needed to examine care in other contexts and to understand how forms and relations of oppression – related to race, ethnicity, and citizenship status – shape processes of renegotiating care responsibilities and imagining alternatives. In my current research project at the University of Calgary, I've been learning from racialized, immigrant women employed in Alberta's long-term care sector about how they navigate and negotiate care responsibilities or find ways to make things work. I'm interested in the different ways they've been set up and summoned, and in the different critical analyses and invitations that follow. I look forward to keeping these conversations going.

So, to close, with a focus on the limits of care, I set out to undertake a disruptive, counter-story-telling project as an artist, critic, and sociologist. On the surface, this book is about how to leave or get out of care work. But, more than that, it's a book about what it means to stay with something. Like a dog with a bone, I've stayed with the trouble, writing with anger and optimism, pushing for something more. Moving forward, I push for alternative ways of organizing and understanding care beyond those that alienate us from ourselves and others or set us up for intimate losses or dilemmas that we spend years confronting. We need ways of loosening care's moral grip or weaning ourselves off care as an all-encompassing ethic, life path, or "only thing." We need tough conversations about what we expect of ourselves and others, about what conditions can help us to thrive, and about how our lives and relationships can be otherwise.

Much like the Care Junkie Recovery Group I had originally envisioned at the start of this project, the stories presented in this book have come to represent a place for caregivers from diverse contexts to gather together. These stories prompt us to tell one story to be able to tell the next, to situate and contextualize our stories in conversation with others, to imagine and push for something more.

I'll set out the coffee and doughnuts.

Appendix 1: Care Junkie Recovery Group – Reading Guide

Reading Guide for Chapter 1, "Care Junkie Diaries: The Memoir"

This book underscores the power of storytelling and conversations in shifting how we understand ourselves and our relationships. The memoir in particular was written to activate a self-reflection process for you and other readers. Whether you are reading this "Care Junkie Recovery Group" guide alone or as part of a group, consider setting a timer for five or ten minutes to free-write in response to questions *that spark something for you*. Write what comes to mind and without overthinking or second-guessing yourself. Remember writing is a way of thinking.

1. What stories from the memoir most stick with you? What stories or insights *came to mind for you* as you read?
2. Janna writes about her experiences as a six-foot-three working-class white woman who entered paid care work in her twenties. What stands out to you about how race, class, gender, and age matter in her care work story? How about in the stories of others you know?
3. In addition to the work of supporting people directly, the memoir mentions other forms of work or ways care providers took responsibility or found self-worth and purpose (in ways that bound them to the work and made it hard to leave). What were some of the joyful or meaningful parts of care work for Janna and her co-workers? Do you agree that care relationships can be sites of transformation? Have you experienced that at all?
4. How would you describe the group home in comparison to L'Arche? How did the working conditions or cultures vary? Do you think those workplaces would be different now than they were in the early 2010s? Do you think young workers have

different ideas about what the work will offer them or about how they should inhabit the role?

5. In what ways do Janna and her co-workers renegotiate, resist, or make meanings of their experiences? Do you think they ever push it too far with some of their critiques? Do you see any value in comparing the struggles of care workers with women experiencing other forms of gender-based violence?

6. As a counter story, the memoir engages head-on with expectations around women's selflessness, secrecy, and limited self-expression in the context of care, as well as with dominant power dynamics that position care providers in relation to others, including managers, people who rely on care, and elite women complimenting them for being "angels." What dominant cultural ideals, work/organizational structures, or ways of coming to inhabit the role made care work difficult for Janna? Do you see any commonalities between paid care staff and unpaid family caregivers at all?

7. In the section titled "Daddy Loves You," Janna introduces a comment from her friend Catherine, who said to her, "The revulsion you experienced speaks to the obscenity of the set up." What do you think was meant by that? Have you had an experience where your sense of what something was about – or what it meant to you – changed dramatically overtime? How about an experience of learning from anger or another emotion as a signal that something needed to change?

8. Janna writes about projecting onto others, struggling to see past her own pain, and otherwise becoming "turned in" on herself and her experience as a care worker. There was a lot getting in the way of her being able to find common ground with others or notice the structural forces at play. What would you say to a care provider who is struggling in their work or feels like a "bad apple" or a "failure"? What questions could you ask them about their situation that might help them to gain more perspective or foster more compassion for themselves?

9. Janna reflects on meaningful conversations with friends and colleagues, and on encounters with scholarly and artistic works, that helped her to critically reflect on her circumstances. Have you had an experience reading or learning something that has shifted your perspective? Anything validating, healing or liberatory?

10. What are the possibilities and limits of memoir-writing or counter-story-telling work for sociology, or life in general? Have you had any experiences using art, critical thinking, or humour as forms of resistance?

11. Okay, so, what pisses *you* off?
12. No, *really*, what pisses you off? Are there any dominant, hegemonic, or common-sense understandings that you've been rethinking in the context of your own life and relationships? For instance, is there a question (like "What's for dinner?" or "Are you dating anyone?") that you're sick and tired of being asked? Is there something that bothers you that you'd be interested in conducting research on? Is there a topic you think would be worth hosting a future recovery group to explore?

Appendix 2: Overview of Participants and Interview Process

I conducted 43 hours and 15 minutes of recorded interviews; this involved meeting with most participants at least once (with each interview averaging an hour and a half). I completed two in-person interviews with Betty (2 hours and 37 minutes total), one in-person interview with Rhonda (1 hour and 40 minutes total), two in-person interviews with Judy (3 hours and 25 minutes total), one in-person and one phone interview with Marilyn (2 hours and 20 minutes total), one in-person interview with Sheila (1 hour and 30 minutes total), two phone interviews with Gina (5 hours and 16 minutes total), two phone interviews with Vicki (3 hours and 2 minutes total), three phone interviews with Gracie (8 hours and 23 minutes total), one in-person interview with Anne (1 hour and 57 minutes total), two in-person interviews with Carrie (3 hours and 53 minutes total), two phone interviews with Nora (4 hours and 2 minutes total), three phone interviews with Troy (7 hours and 56 minutes total), and one phone interview with Julie (1 hour and 54 minutes total). The shortest interview was 53 minutes (my second meeting with Marilyn), and the longest interview was 3 hours and 9 minutes (my third meeting with Gracie).

Table 1. Overview of Participants

Name	Age Cohort	Ethnicity	Family Ties	Class Position and Resources	Work/Care Experiences
Betty	World War II (b. 1940s)	Indigenous	Married with three children	High-income professional-class household	Late-life family carer (for husband), retired public servant, and former teacher
Rhonda	World War II (b. 1940s)	White	Single with three children	Moderate-income professional-class household	Former late-life family carer (for late husband), retired mental health nurse
Judy	World War II (b. 1940s)	White	Single with two children	Moderate-income household	Former late-life family carer (for late husband and parents), retired secretary
Marilyn	World War II (b. 1940s)	White	Married with two children	High-income professional-class household	Former late-life family carer (for parents), retired nurse
Sheila	Baby boomer (b. 1950s)	White	Married with two children	High-income professional-class household	Former family carer (for mother), retired government director
Vicki	Baby boomer (b. 1950s)	White	Single with no children	Moderate-income professional-class household	AIDS activist and former care team member, retired professional
Gina	Baby boomer (b. 1950s)	White	Divorced with two children	Low-income working-class household	Former family carer (for mother), former home day-care operator
Gracie	Baby boomer (b. 1960s)	White	Married with two children	Moderate-income working-class household	Former family carer (for mother, husband, children), former home day-care operator, administrative assistant

(*Continued*)

Table 1. (Continued)

Name	Age Cohort	Ethnicity	Family Ties	Class Position and Resources	Work/Care Experiences
Anne	Baby boomer (b. ?1960s)	White	Married with two children	Moderate-income professional-class household	Family carer (for disabled child), professional
Carrie	Millennial (b. 1980s)	Indigenous	Single with two children	Low-income working-class household	Former homeless service centre worker, doula
Nora	Millennial (b. 1980s)	White	Partnered with no children	Low-income professional-class household	Former support worker at residential group home
Troy	Millennial (b. 1980s)	White	Single with no children	Low-income professional-class household	Former homeless service centre worker
Julie	Millennial (b. 1990s)	White	Single with no children	Moderate-income professional-class household	Former live-in assistant at L'Arche, professional

References

Abel, Emily K. 2000. "A Historical Perspective on Care." In *Care Work: Gender, Labor, and the Welfare State*, edited by Madonna Harrington Meyer, 8–14. New York: Routledge.

Addati, Laura, Umberto Cattaneo, Valeria Esquivel, and Isabel Valarino. 2018. *Care Work and Care Jobs for the Future of Decent Work*. International Labour Organisation (ILO).

Ahmed, Sara. 2020. "Feminists at Work." *feministkilljoys*, 10 January. https:// feministkilljoys.com/2020/01/10/feminists-at-work/.

Andrews, Molly. 2004. "Opening to the Original Contributions." In *Considering Counter-Narratives: Narrating, Resisting, Making Sense*, edited by Michael Bamberg and Molly Andrews, 1–7. Amsterdam: John Benjamins.

Armstrong, Pat. 2007. "Back to Basics: Seeking Pay Equity for Women in Canada." *Labour & Industry: A Journal of the Social and Economic Relations of Work* 18 (2): 11–32. https://doi.org/10.1080/10301763.2007.10669363.

– 2013. "Puzzling Skills: Feminist Political Economy Approaches." *Canadian Review of Sociology* 50 (3): 256–83. https://doi.org/10.1111/cars.12015.

–, ed. 2023. *Unpaid Work in Nursing Homes: Flexible Boundaries*. Bristol, UK: Policy Press.

Armstrong, Pat, and Hugh Armstrong, eds. 2019. *The Privatization of Care: The Case of Nursing Homes*. New York: Routledge.

Armstrong, Pat, Hugh Armstrong, Jacqueline Choiniere, Ruth Lowndes, and James Struthers. 2020. *Re-imagining Long-Term Residential Care in the COVID-19 Crisis*. Ottawa: Canadian Centre for Policy Alternatives.

Armstrong, Pat, Albert Banerjee, Hugh Armstrong, Susan Braedley, Jacqueline Choiniere, Ruth Lowndes, and Jim Struthers. 2019. *Models for Long-Term Residential Care: A Summary of the Consultants' Report to Long-Term Care Homes and Services, City of Toronto*. https://www.toronto.ca/legdocs/mmis/2019 /ec/bgrd/backgroundfile-130891.pdf.

Armstrong, Pat, Albert Banerjee, Marta Szebehely, Hugh Armstrong, Tamara Daly, and Stirling Lafrance. 2009. *They Deserve Better. The Long-Term Care Experience in Canada and Scandinavia*. Ottawa: The Canadian Centre for Policy Alternatives.

Armstrong, Pat, and Susan Braedley, eds. 2013. *Troubling Care: Critical Perspectives on Research and Practices*. Toronto: Canadian Scholars.

–, eds. 2023. *Care Homes in a Turbulent Era: Do They Have a Future?* Cheltenham, UK: Edward Elgar.

Armstrong, Pat, and Janna Klostermann. 2023. "Unpaid Care in Public Places: Tensions in Times of Covid-19." In *From Crisis to Catastrophe: Care, COVID, and Pathways to Change,* edited by Mignon Duffy, Amy Armenia, and Kim Price-Glynn, 53–60. New Brunswick, NJ: Rutgers University Press.

Aronson, Jane. 1998. "Dutiful Daughters and Undemanding Mothers: Constraining Images of Giving and Receiving Care in Middle and Later Life." In *Women's Caring: Feminist Perspectives on Social Welfare* (2nd ed.), edited by Carol T. Baines, Patricia Evans, and Sheila M. Neysmith, 114–38. Toronto: Oxford University Press.

– 2002. "Elderly People's Accounts of Home Care Rationing: Missing Voices in Long-term Care Policy Debates." *Ageing & Society* 22 (4): 399–418. https://pubmed.ncbi.nlm.nih.gov/15264341/. Medline:15264341

Baines, Donna. 2004. "Caring for Nothing: Work Organization and Unwaged Labour in Social Services." *Work, Employment and Society* 18 (2): 267–95. https://doi.org/10.1177/09500172004042770.

– 2015. "Neoliberalism and the Convergence of Nonprofit Care Work in Canada." *Competition & Change* 19 (3): 194–209. https://doi.org/10.1177/1024529415580258.

Baines, Donna, and Pat Armstrong. 2019. "Non-Job Work/Unpaid Caring: Gendered Industrial Relations in Long-Term Care." *Gender, Work & Organization* 26 (7): 934–47. https://doi.org/10.1111/gwao.12293.

Baines, Donna, Susan Braedley, Tamara Daly, et al. 2024. "But Where's the Body? Bodies, Time, Money, and the Political Economy of Post-Pandemic Field Research." *Qualitative Research*, ahead of print, 7 August. https://doi.org/10.1177/14687941241264473.

Baines, Donna, and Tamara Daly. 2015. "Resisting Regulatory Rigidities: Lessons from Front-Line Care Work." *Studies in Political Economy* 95 (1): 137–160. https://doi.org/10.1080/19187033.2015.11674949.

Baines, Donna, Paul Kent, and Sally Kent. 2019. "'Off My Own Back': Precarity on the Frontlines of Care Work." *Work, Employment and Society* 33 (5): 877–87. https://doi.org/10.1177/0950017018817488.

Banerjee, Albert, Tamara Daly, Pat Armstrong, Marta Szebehely, Hugh Armstrong, and Stirling Lafrance. 2012. "Structural Violence in Long-Term Residential Care for Older People: Comparing Canada and Scandinavia."

Social Science & Medicine 74 (3): 390–8. https://doi.org/10.1016/j.socscimed
.2011.10.037. Medline:22204839

Barad, Karen. 2007. *Meeting the Universe Halfway: Quantum Physics and the
Entanglement of Matter and Meaning.* Durham, NC: Duke University Press.

Barnett, Jenna. 2023. "What Is Spiritual Abuse? And How Do We Heal from
It?" *Sojourners*, 10 August. https://sojo.net/articles/what-spiritual-abuse
-church-and-how-do-we-heal-it.

Basting, Anne. 2020. *Creative Care: A Revolutionary Approach to Dementia and
Elder Care.* New York: Harper One.

Ben-Ahmed, Houssem Eddine, and Ivy Lynn Bourgeault. 2023. "Sustaining
the Canadian Nursing Workforce: Targeted Evidence-Based Reactive
Solutions in Response to the Ongoing Crisis." *Nursing Leadership* 35 (4):
14–29. https://doi.org/10.12927/cjnl.2023.27076. Medline:37216294

Bernikow, Louise. 1980. *Among Women.* New York: Harmony Books.

Beverley, Andrea. 2011. "Grounds for Telling It: Transnational Feminism and
Canadian Women's Writing." PhD diss., Université de Montréal. https://
hdl.handle.net/1866/4843.

Bezanson, Kate, and Meg Luxton. 2006. *Social Reproduction: Feminist Political
Economy Challenges Neo-Liberalism.* Montreal: McGill-Queen's University Press.

Black, Simon. 2020. *Social Reproduction and the City: Welfare Reform, Child Care,
and Resistance in Neoliberal New York.* Athens, GA: University of Georgia Press.

Blix, Bodil H., Vera Caine, D. Jean Clandinin, and Charlotte Berendonk. 2021.
"Considering Silences in Narrative Inquiry: An Intergenerational Story of
a Sami Family." *Journal of Contemporary Ethnography* 50 (4): 580–94. https://
doi.org/10.1177/08912416211003145.

Block, Sheila, and Grace-Edward Galabuzi. 2011. *Canada's Colour Coded Labour
Market: The Gap for Racialized Workers.* Ottawa: Canadian Centre for Policy
Alternatives.

Bordo, Susan. 2003. *Unbearable Weight: Feminism, Western Culture, and the Body.*
10th anniversary ed. Berkeley: University of California Press.

Braedley, Susan. 2013. "A Gender Politics of Long-Term Care: Towards an
Analysis." In *Troubling Care: Critical Perspectives on Research and Practices,*
edited by Pat Armstrong and Susan Braedley, 59–70. Toronto: Canadian
Scholars.

– 2015. "Pulling Men into the Care Economy: The Case of Canadian
Firefighters." *Competition & Change* 19 (3): 264–78. https://doi.org/10.1177
/1024529415580259.

– 2018. "Reinventing the Nursing Home: Metaphors that Design Care." In
Ageing in Everyday Life: Materialities and Embodiments, edited by Stephen
Katz, 45–63. Bristol, UK: Policy Press.

Braedley, Susan, Pat Armstrong, and Janna Klostermann. 2023. "Making Joy
Possible in Care Home Policies and Practices." In *Care Homes in a Turbulent*

Era: Do They Have A Future?, edited by Pat Armstrong and Susan Braedley, 151–68. Cheltenham, UK: Edward Elgar.

Braedley, Susan, Karine Côté-Boucher, and Anna Przednowek. 2021. "Old and Dangerous: Bordering Older Migrants' Mobilities, Rejuvenating the Post-Welfare State." *Social Politics: International Studies in Gender, State & Society* 28 (1): 24–46. https://doi.org/10.1093/sp/jxz028.

Braedley, Susan, and Meg Luxton. 2021. "Social Reproduction at Work, Social Reproduction as Work: A Feminist Political Economy Perspective." *Journal of Labor and Society* 25 (4): 559–86. https://doi.org/10.1163/24714607-bja10049.

Braedley, Susan, Prince Owusu, Anna Przednowek, and Pat Armstrong. 2018. "We're Told, 'Suck It Up': Long-Term Care Workers' Psychological Health and Safety." *Ageing International* 43 (1): 91–109. https://doi.org/10.1007/s12126-017-9288-4.

Brassolotto, Julia, Lisa Howard, and Alessandro Manduca-Barone. 2020. "'If You Do Not Find the World Tasty and Sexy, You Are Out of Touch with the Most Important Things in Life': Resident and Family Member Perspectives on Sexual Expression in Continuing Care." *Journal of Aging Studies* 53 (100849). https://doi.org/10.1016/j.jaging.2020.100849. Medline:32487340

Brickell, Chris. 2003. "Performativity or Performance? Clarifications in the Sociology of Gender." *New Zealand Sociology* 18 (2): 158–78.

Bryant, Joanne, and Toni Schofield. 2007. "Feminine Sexual Subjectivities: Bodies, Agency and Life History." *Sexualities* 10 (3): 321–40. https://doi.org/10.1177/1363460707078321.

Byrne, Bridget. 2006. "In Search of a 'Good Mix': 'Race,' Class, Gender and Practices of Mothering." *Sociology* 40 (6): 1001–17. https://doi.org/10.1177/0038038506069841.

Caputo, John D., ed. 1997. *Deconstruction in a Nutshell: A Conversation with Jacques Derrida*. New York: Fordham University Press.

Carrier-Moisan, Marie-Eve. 2014. "Saving Women? Awkward Alliances in the Public Spaces of Sex Tourism." In *Contesting Publics: Feminism, Activism, Ethnography*, edited by Lynne Phillips, Sally Cole, Marie-Eve Carrier-Moisan, Erica Lagalisse, Vered Amit, and Jon P. Mitchell, 48–75. London: Pluto Press.

– 2015. "'Putting Femininity to Work': Negotiating Hypersexuality and Respectability in Sex Tourism, Brazil." *Sexualities* 18 (4): 499–518. https://doi.org/10.1177/1363460714550902.

– 2020. *Gringo Love: Stories of Sex Tourism in Brazil*. Toronto: University of Toronto Press.

Cerwonka, Allaine, and Liisa H. Malkki. 2008. *Improvising Theory: Process and Temporality in Ethnographic Fieldwork*. Chicago: University of Chicago Press.

"Charlottetown Declaration on the Right to Care." 2001. https://thecareeconomy.ca/wp-content/uploads/2021/09/Charlottetown-Declaration.pdf.

Chivers, Sally. 2013. "Care, Culture and Creativity: A Disability Perspective on Long-Term Residential Care." In *Troubling Care: Critical Perspectives on Research and Practices*, edited by Pat Armstrong and Susan Braedley, 47–58. Toronto: Canadian Scholars.

– 2020. "Cripping Care Advice." In *The Aging–Disability Nexus*, edited by Katie Aubrecht, Christine Kelly, and Carla Rice, 51–64. Vancouver: UBC Press.

– 2021. "Old Friends: Reimagining Care Relations Through Helen Garner's *The Spare Room*." In *Contemporary Narratives of Ageing, Illness, Care*, edited by Katsura Sako and Sarah Falcus, 163–76. New York: Routledge.

– 2023. "Home Care, Cinema, and the Relational Turn in Age Studies." In *The Bloomsbury Handbook to Ageing in Contemporary Literature and Film*, edited by Sarah Falcus, Heike Hartung, and Raquel Medina Bañón, 213–23. London: Bloomsbury.

Chivers, Sally, and Ulla Kriebernegg. 2017. *Care Home Stories: Aging, Disability, and Long-Term Residential Care*. Bielefeld, Germany: Transcript Verlag.

Chun, Jennifer J., and Cynthia Cranford. 2018. "Becoming Homecare Workers: Chinese Immigrant Women and the Changing Worlds of Work, Care and Unionism." *Critical Sociology* 44 (7–8): 1013–27. https://doi.org/10.1177/0896920517748499.

Clifford Simplican, Stacy. 2015. "Care, Disability, and Violence: Theorizing Complex Dependency in Eva Kittay and Judith Butler." *Hypatia* 30 (1): 217–33. https://www.jstor.org/stable/24542068.

Code, Lorraine. 2006. *Ecological Thinking: The Politics of Epistemic Location*. Oxford: Oxford University Press.

– 2020. *Manufactured Uncertainty: Implications for Climate Change Skepticism*. New York: SUNY Press.

Cohen, Stanley. 1980. *Folk Devils and Moral Panics: The Creation of the Mods and Rockers*. New York: Martin Roberston.

Cole, Sally, Marie-Eve Carrier-Moisan, Erica Lagalisse, and Lynne Phillips. 2014. "A Pedagogical Conversation: Public Scholars and Public Scholarship." In *Contesting Publics: Feminism, Activism, Ethnography*, edited by Lynne Phillips, Sally Cole, Marie-Eve Carrier-Moisan, Erica Lagalisse, Vered Amit, and Jon P. Mitchell, 138–48. London: Pluto Press.

Connell, Raewyn. 2000. *The Men and the Boys*. Berkeley: University of California Press.

– 2002. *Gender*. Cambridge, UK: Polity Press.

– 2005. *Masculinities* (2nd ed.). Berkeley: University of California Press.

– 2012. "Transsexual Women and Feminist Thought: Toward New Understanding and New Politics." *Signs: Journal of Women in Culture and Society* 37 (4): 857–81. https://doi.org/10.1086/664478.

Corley, Mary C., Ptlene Minick, R.K. Elswick, and Mary Jacobs. 2005. "Nurse Moral Distress and Ethical Work Environment." *Nursing Ethics* 12 (4): 381–90. https://doi.org/10.1191/0969733005ne809oa. Medline:16045246

Côté-Boucher, Karine, Tamara Daly, Sally Chivers, Susan Braedley, and Sean Hillier. 2024. "Counter-Narratives of Active Aging: Disability, Trauma, and Joy in the Age-Friendly City." *Journal of Aging Studies* 68: 101205. https://doi.org/10.1016/j.jaging.2023.101205. Medline:38458724

Cranford, Cynthia. 2020. *Home Care Fault Lines: Understanding Tensions and Creating Alliances*. Ithaca, NY: Cornell University Press.

Cvetkovich, Ann. 2012. *Depression: A Public Feeling*. Durham, NC: Duke University Press.

Daly, Tamara. 2015. "Dancing the Two-Step in Ontario's Long-Term Care Sector: Deterrence Regulation = Consolidation." *Studies in Political Economy* 95 (1): 29–58. https://doi.org/10.1080/19187033.2015.11674945.

Daly, Tamara, and Marta Szebehely. 2012. "Unheard Voices, Unmapped Terrain: Care Work in Long-Term Residential Care for Older People in Canada and Sweden." *International Journal of Social Welfare* 21 (2): 139–48. https://doi.org/10.1111/j.1468-2397.2011.00806.x. Medline:24999303

Das Gupta, Tania. 2020. "Inquiry into Coronavirus Nursing Home Deaths Needs to Include Discussion of Workers and Race." *The Conversation*, 25 May. https://theconversation.com/inquiry-into-coronavirus-nursing-home-deaths-needs-to-include-discussion-of-workers-and-race-139017.

Davidson, Rachel Diana. 2015. "Rhetorical Lessons in Advocacy and Shared Responsibility: Family Metaphors and Definitions of Crisis and Care in Unpaid Family Caregiving Advocacy Rhetoric." PhD diss., University of Wisconsin-Milwaukee. https://dc.uwm.edu/etd/994/.

Day, Suzanne. 2013. "The Implications of Conceptualizing Care." In *Troubling Care: Critical Perspectives on Research and Practices*, edited by Pat Armstrong and Susan Braedley, 21–32. Toronto: Canadian Scholars.

Delitala, Albert. 2020. "Coronavirus: Markham, Ont., Care Home Taking Applications amid Staffing Shortage, COVID-19 Outbreak." *Global News*, 11 April. https://globalnews.ca/news/6808596/coronavirus-markham-care-home-jobs-covid-19/.

Devi, Reena, Claire Goodman, Sonia Dalkin, et al. 2021. "Attracting, Recruiting and Retaining Nurses and Care Workers Working in Care Homes: The Need for a Nuanced Understanding Informed by Evidence and Theory." *Age and Ageing* 50 (1): 65–7. https://doi.org/10.1093/ageing/afaa109. Medline:32614968

Dodson, Lisa, and Wendy Luttrell. 2011. "Families Facing Untenable Choices." *Contexts* 10 (1): 38–42. https://doi.org/10.1177/1536504211399049.

Donath, Orna. 2015. "Regretting Motherhood: A Sociopolitical Analysis." *Signs: Journal of Women in Culture and Society* 40 (2): 343–67. https://doi.org/10.1086/678145.

Dosekun, Simidele. 2020. *Fashioning Postfeminism: Spectacular Femininity and Transnational Culture*. Urbana: University of Illinois Press.

Doucet, Andrea. 2006. *Do Men Mother? Fathering, Care, and Domestic Responsibility*. Toronto: University of Toronto Press.

– 2018. "Decolonizing Family Photographs: Ecological Imaginaries and Nonrepresentational Ethnographies." *Journal of Contemporary Ethnography* 47 (6): 729–57. https://doi.org/10.1177/0891241617744859.

– 2020. "Father Involvement, Care, and Breadwinning: Genealogies of Concepts and Revisioned Conceptual Narratives." *Genealogy* 4 (1): 1–17. https://doi.org/10.3390/genealogy4010014.

– 2021. "What Does Rachel Carson Have to Do with Family Sociology and Family Policies? Ecological Imaginaries, Relational Ontologies, and Crossing Social Imaginaries." *Families, Relationships and Societies*, 10 (1): 11–31. https://doi.org/10.1332/204674321X16111320274832.

– 2022. "'Time Is Not Time Is Not Time': A Feminist Ecological Approach to Clock Time, Process Time, and Care Responsibilities." *Time & Society* 32 (4): 434–60. https://doi.org/10.1177/0961463X221133894.

Doucet, Andrea, and Janna Klostermann. 2023. "What and How Are We Measuring When We Research Gendered Divisions of Domestic Labour? Remaking the Household Portrait as Method into a Care/Work Portrait. " *Sociological Research Online* 29 (1): 243–63. https://doi.org/10.1177/13607804231160740.

Doucet, Andrea, and Natasha S. Mauthner. 2008. "What Can Be Known and How? Narrated Subjects and the Listening Guide." *Qualitative Research* 8 (3): 399–409. https://doi.org/10.1177/1468794106093636.

Duffy, Mignon. 2005. "Reproducing Labor Inequalities: Challenges for Feminists Conceptualizing Care at the Intersections of Gender, Race, and Class." *Gender & Society* 19 (1): 66–82. https://doi.org/10.1177/0891243204269499.

– 2011. *Making Care Count: A Century of Gender, Race, and Paid Care Work*. New Brunswick, NJ: Rutgers University Press.

Duffy, Mignon, Amy Armenia, and Clare L. Stacey, eds. 2015. *Caring on the Clock: The Complexities and Contradictions of Paid Care Work*. New Brunswick, NJ: Rutgers University Press.

Eicher-Catt, Deborah. 2005. "The Myth of Servant-Leadership: A Feminist Perspective." *Women & Language* 28 (1): 17.

Eiesland, Nancy L. 1994. *The Disabled God: Toward a Liberatory Theology of Disability*. Nashville: Abingdon Press.

Ellingson, Laura L. 2017. *Embodiment in Qualitative Research*. New York: Routledge.

Eltahawy, Mona. 2019. *The Seven Necessary Sins for Women and Girls*. Boston: Beacon Press.

England, Kim, and Isabel Dyck. 2011. "Managing the Body Work of Home Care." *Sociology of Health & Illness* 33 (2): 206–19. https://doi.org/10.1111/j.1467-9566.2010.01331.x. Medline:21299569

Ezawa, Aya. 2016. *Single Mothers in Contemporary Japan: Motherhood, Class, and Reproductive Practice*. Lanham, MD: Lexington Books.

Ezawa, Aya, and Chisa Fujiwara. 2005. "Lone Mothers and Welfare-to-Work Policies in Japan and the United States: Toward an Alternative Perspective." *Journal of Sociology & Social Welfare* 32 (4): 41–63. https://doi.org/10.15453 /0191-5096.3113.

Federici, Silvia. 2012. *Revolution at Point Zero: Housework, Reproduction, and Feminist Struggle*. Oakland, CA: PM Press.

Ferguson, Susan. 2008. "Canadian Contributions to Social Reproduction Feminism, Race and Embodied Labor." *Race, Gender & Class* 15 (1–2): 42–57. https://www.jstor.org/stable/41675357.

Finch, Janet, and Jennifer Mason. 1992. *Negotiating Family Responsibilities*. London: Routledge.

FitzGerald, Maggie. 2020. "Aging, Disability, and Long-Term-Care Policy." In *The Aging–Disability Nexus*, edited by Katie Aubrecht, Christine Kelly, and Carla Rice, 83–96. Vancouver: UBC Press.

Folbre, Nancy, Shawn Fremstad, Pilar Gonalons-Pons, and Victoria Coan. 2023. "Measuring Care Provision in the United States: Resources, Shortfalls, and Possible Improvements." Working Paper. Center for Economic Policy Research.

Folbre, Nancy, Leila Gautham, and Kristin Smith. 2021. "Essential Workers and Care Penalties in the United States." *Feminist Economics* 27 (1–2): 173–87. https://doi.org/10.1080/13545701.2020.1828602.

Forna, Aminatta. 1999. *Mother of all Myths: How Society Moulds and Constrains Mothers*. London: Harper Collins.

Frank, Arthur W. 2010. *Letting Stories Breathe: A Socio-Narratology*. Chicago: University of Chicago Press.

Fraser, Nancy. 2016. "Contradictions of Capital and Care." *New Left Review* 100 (July/Aug): 99–117.

Fraser, Nancy, and Linda Gordon. 1994. "A Genealogy of Dependency: Tracing a Keyword of the US Welfare State." *Signs: Journal of Women in Culture and Society* 19 (2): 309–36. https://www.jstor.org/stable/3174801.

Freire, Paulo. 1972. *Pedagogy of the Oppressed*. Translated by Myra Bergman Ramos. New York: Herder & Herder.

Funk, Laura. 2015. "Constructing the Meaning of Filial Responsibility: Choice and Obligation in the Accounts of Adult Children." *Families, Relationships and Societies* 4 (3): 383–99. https://doi.org/10.1332/20467431 4X14110461145506.

Funk, Laura M., Rachel Herron, Dale Spencer, Lisette Dansereau, and Megan Wrathall. 2019. "More Than 'Petty Squabbles': Developing a Contextual Understanding of Conflict and Aggression among Older Women in Low-Income Assisted Living." *Journal of Aging Studies* 48: 1–8. https://doi.org /10.1016/j.jaging.2018.11.001.

Funk, Laura M., Janna Klostermann, Holly Symonds-Brown, Katie Aubrecht, and Lauriane Giguère. 2024. "Producing the Public Caregiver: The Discursive Politicization of Family Caregiving by Canadian Caregiver Organizations." *International Journal of Care and Caring*, ahead of print, 16 September. https://doi.org/10.1332/23978821Y2024D000000079.

Funk, Laura M., and Linda Outcalt. 2019. "Maintaining the 'Caring Self' and Working Relationships: A Critically Informed Analysis of Meaning-Construction among Paid Companions in Long-Term Residential Care." *Ageing & Society* 40 (7): 1511–28. https://doi.org/10.1017/S0144686X19000138.

Gardiner Barber, Pauline. 2000. "Agency in Philippine Women's Labour Migration and Provisional Diaspora." *Women's Studies International Forum* 23 (4): 399–411. https://doi.org/10.1016/S0277-5395(00)00104-7.

Garland-Thomson, Rosemarie. 2007. "Shape Structures Story: Fresh and Feisty Stories about Disability." *Narrative* 15 (1): 113–23. http://doi.org/10.1353/nar.2007.0005.

– 2017. "Julia Pastrana, the 'Extraordinary Lady.'" *Alter* 11 (1): 35–49. https://doi.org/10.1016/j.alter.2016.12.001.

Gilchrist, Karen. 2021. "Covid Has Made It Harder to Be a Health-Care Worker. Now, Many Are Thinking of Quitting." *CNBC*, 30 May. https://www.cnbc.com/2021/05/31/covid-is-driving-an-exodus-among-health-care-workers.html.

Gill-Austern, Brita L. 1996. "Love Understood as Self-Sacrifice and Self-Denial: What Does It Do to Women?" In *Through the Eyes of Women*, edited by Jeanne Stevenson Moessner, 304–21. Minneapolis, MN: Fortress Press.

Gilligan, Carol. 1982. *In a Different Voice: Psychological Theory and Women's Development*. Cambridge, MA: Harvard University Press.

Glenn, Evelyn Nakano. 2010. *Forced to Care: Coercion and Caregiving in America*. Cambridge, MA: Harvard University Press.

Goodson, Ivor F. 1992. "Studying Teachers' Lives: An Emergent Field of Inquiry." In *Studying Teachers' Lives*, edited by Ivor F. Goodson, 1–17. London: Routledge.

Gottfried, Heidi, and Jennifer Jihye Chun. 2018. "Care Work in Transition: Transnational Circuits of Gender, Migration, and Care." *Critical Sociology* 44(7–8): 997–1012. https://doi.org/10.1177/0896920518765931.

Grenier, Amanda, Meredith Griffin, and Colleen McGrath. 2020. "Aging and Disability: The Paradoxical Positions of the Chronological Life Course." In *The Aging–Disability Nexus*, edited by Katie Aubrecht, Christine Kelly, and Carla Rice, 21–34. Vancouver: UBC Press.

Grey Jillian M., Vasiliki Totsika, and Richard P. Hastings. 2018. "Physical and Psychological Health of Family Carers Co-Residing with an Adult Relative with an Intellectual Disability." *Journal of Applied Research in Intellectual Disabilities* 31 (S2): 191–202. https://doi.org/10.1111/jar.12353. Medline:28378391

Grigorovich, Alisa, and Pia Kontos. 2019. "A Critical Realist Exploration of the Vulnerability of Staff to Sexual Harassment in Residential Long-Term Care." *Social Science & Medicine*. 238 (112356). https://doi.org/10.1016/j.socscimed.2019.112356. Medline:31204030

Hartman, Saidiya. 2008. *Lose Your Mother: A Journey Along the Atlantic Slave Route*. New York: Farrar, Straus and Giroux.

Hendriks, Ruud. 2012. "Tackling Indifference: Clowning, Dementia, and the Articulation of a Sensitive Body." *Medical Anthropology* 31 (6): 459–76. https://doi.org/10.1080/01459740.2012.674991. Medline:22985107

Herron, Rachel V., Laura Funk, and Dale Spencer. 2019. "Responding the 'Wrong Way': The Emotion Work of Caring for a Family Member with Dementia." *Gerontologist* 59 (5): 470–8. https://doi.org/10.1093/geront/gnz047. Medline:31050725

Hollway, Wendy. 2006. *The Capacity to Care: Gender and Ethical Subjectivity*. London: Routledge.

Irving, Dan. 2017. "Gender Transition and Job In/Security: Trans* Un/der/ employment Experiences and Labour Anxieties in Post-Fordist Society." *Atlantis: Critical Studies in Gender, Culture & Social Justice* 38 (1): 168–78. https://atlantisjournal.ca/index.php/atlantis/article/view/4778.

Joseph, Alun E., and Mark W. Skinner. 2012. "Voluntarism as a Mediator of the Experience of Growing Old in Evolving Rural Spaces and Changing Rural Places." *Journal of Rural Studies* 28 (4): 380–8. https://doi.org/10.1016/j.jrurstud.2012.01.007.

Katz, Stephen. 2017. "Generation X: A Critical Sociological Perspective." *Generations* 41 (3): 12–19. https://www.jstor.org/stable/26556295.

Kearney, Tim, ed. 2000. *A Prophetic Cry: Stories of Spirituality and Healing Inspired by L'Arche*. Dublin: Veritas.

Keleta-Mae, Naila. 2023. *Performing Female Blackness*. Waterloo, ON: Wilfrid Laurier University Press.

Kelly, Brighid. 1998. "Preserving Moral Integrity: A Follow-Up Study with New Graduate Nurses." *Journal of Advanced Nursing* 28 (5): 1134–45. https://doi.org/10.1046/j.1365-2648.1998.00810.x. Medline:9840887

Kennelly, Jacqueline. 2014. "'It's This Pain in My Heart That Won't Let Me Stop': Gendered Affect, Webs of Relations, and Young Women's Activism." *Feminist Theory* 15 (3): 241–60. https://doi.org/10.1177/1464700114544611.

Kim, Yang-Sook. 2018. "Care Work and Ethnic Boundary Marking in South Korea." *Critical Sociology* 44 (7–8): 1045–59. https://doi.org/10.1177/0896920518766397.

King, Andrew, and Ann Cronin. 2013. "Queering Care in Later Life: The Lived Experiences and Intimacies of Older Lesbian, Gay and Bisexual Adults." In *Mapping Intimacies: Relations, Exchanges, Affects*, edited by Tam Sanger and Yvette Taylor, 112–29. London: Palgrave Macmillan.

Kittay, Eva Feder. 1999. *Love's Labor: Essays on Women, Equality, and Dependency*. New York: Routledge.

Klostermann, Janna. 2019. "Altering Imaginaries and Demanding Treatment: Women's AIDS Activism in Toronto, 1980s–1990s." In *Women's Health Advocacy: Rhetorical Ingenuity for the 21st Century*, edited by Jamie White-Farnham, Bryna Siegel Finer, and Cathryn Molloy, 177–90. New York: Routledge.

– 2020. "Opinion: L'Arche International Has a History of Exploiting Women." *Toronto Star*, 2 March. https://www.thestar.com/opinion /contributors/2020/03/02/larche-international-has-a-history-of-exploiting -women.html.

– 2021. "Care Has Limits: Women's Moral Lives and Revised Meanings of Care." PhD diss., Carleton University. https://doi.org/10.22215/etd/2021 -14352.

– 2023. "Bev Said 'No': Learning from Nursing Home Residents about Care Politics in our Aging Society." *The Gerontologist* 63 (10): 1663–71. https:// doi.org/10.1093/geront/gnad069. Medline:37330624

Klostermann, Janna, Saro Bunting, Krys Maki, and Anna Przednowek. 2025. "Care Containers: The Multi-Layered Politics of Boundless Work in Canada's Victim Services Sector." *Studies in Political Economy*.

Klostermann, Janna, and Lara Funk. 2022. "More Than a Visitor? Rethinking Metaphors for Family Care in Long-Term Care Homes." *Ageing & Society*, ahead of print, 24 November. https://doi.org/10.1017/S0144686X22001271.

– 2024. "Bounding the Boundless: Gendered Work Hierarchies and 'Boundless Work' in Ontario Long-Term Care Homes." *Studies in Political Economy*.

Klostermann, Janna, Laura Funk, Holly Symonds-Brown, et al. 2022. "The Problems with Care: A Feminist Care Scholar Retrospective." *Societies* 12 (2): 52. https://doi.org/10.3390/soc12020052.

Kraus, Chris. 2006. *I Love Dick*. Los Angeles: Semiotext(e).

Ladd-Taylor, Molly. 2004. "Mother-Worship/Mother-Blame: Politics and Welfare in an Uncertain Age." *Journal of the Motherhood Initiative for Research and Community Involvement*, 6 (1): 7–15. https://jarm.journals.yorku.ca /index.php/jarm/article/view/4881.

Lan, Pei-Chia. 2016. "Deferential Surrogates and Professional Others: Recruitment and Training of Migrant Care Workers in Taiwan and Japan." *Positions: Asia Critique* 24 (1): 253–79. https://doi.org/10.1215/10679847-3320137.

Lanoix, Monique. 2005. "No Room for Abuse." *Cultural Studies* 19 (6): 719–36. https://doi.org/10.1080/09502380500365671.

Le Espiritu, Yen. 2001. "'We Don't Sleep Around Like White Girls Do': Family, Culture, and Gender in Filipina American Lives." *Signs: Journal of Women in Culture and Society* 26 (2): 415–40. https://www.jstor.org/stable/3175448.

Levitsky, S.R. 2014. *Caring for Our Own: Why There Is No Political Demand for New American Social Welfare Rights*. New York: Oxford University Press.

Lewis, Camille Kaminski. 2007. *Romancing the Difference: Kenneth Burke, Bob Jones University, and the Rhetoric of Religious Fundamentalism*. Waco, TX: Baylor University Press.

Lightman, Naomi. 2019. "The Migrant in the Market: Care Penalties and Immigration in Eight Liberal Welfare Regimes." *Journal of European Social Policy* 29 (2): 182–96. https://doi.org/10.1177/0958928718768337.

– 2022. "Caring During the COVID-19 Crisis: Intersectional Exclusion of Immigrant Women Health Care Aides in Canadian Long-Term Care." *Health and Social Care in the Community* 30 (4): e1343–51. https://doi.org/10.1111/hsc.13541. Medline:34396607

Lightman, Naomi, and Hamid Akbary. 2023. "Working More and Making Less: Post-Retirement Aged Immigrant Women Care Workers in Canada." *Journal of Aging & Social Policy* 35 (2): 261–86. https://doi.org/10.1080/08959420.2022.2139984. Medline:36682060

Littler, Jo. 2024. "The University: Caring Community or Carewashing Central? Autosociobiographical Reflections." *Educational Philosophy and Theory* 57 (3): 235–47. https://doi.org/10.1080/00131857.2024.2396445.

Lloyd, Liz, Albert Banerjee, Charlene Harrington, Frode F. Jacobsen, and Marta Szebehely. 2014. "It's a Scandal! Comparing the Causes and Consequences of Nursing Home Media Scandals in Five Countries." *International Journal of Sociology and Social Policy* 34 (1/2): 2–18. https://doi.org/10.1108/IJSSP-03-2013-0034.

Lopesi, Lana. 2021. *Bloody Woman: Essays*. Wellington, NZ: Bridget Williams Books.

Lorde, Audre. 2012. *Sister Outsider: Essays and Speeches*. Berkeley, CA: Crossing Press.

Luttrell, Wendy. 2000. "'Good Enough' Methods for Ethnographic Research." *Harvard Educational Review* 70 (4): 499–523.

– 2013. "Children's Counter-Narratives of Care: Towards Educational Justice." *Children & Society* 27 (4): 295–308. http://doi.org/10.1111/chso.12033.

– 2020. *Children Framing Childhoods: Working-Class Kids' Visions of Care*. Bristol, UK: Policy Press.

Luxton, Meg. 1980. *More than a Labour of Love: Three Generations of Women's Work in the Home*. Toronto: Women's Press.

Luxton, Meg, and June Corman. 2001. *Getting By in Hard Times: Gendered Labour at Home and on the Job*. Toronto: University of Toronto Press.

Mahon, Rianne, and Fiona Robinson, eds. 2011. *Feminist Ethics and Social Policy: Towards a New Global Political Economy of Care*. Vancouver: UBC Press.

Mattingly, Cheryl. 2014. *Moral Laboratories: Family Peril and the Struggle for a Good Life*. Berkeley: University of California Press.

McMahon, Martha. 1995. *Engendering Motherhood: Identity and Self-Transformation in Women's Lives*. New York: Guilford Press.

McRobbie, Angela. 1993. "Shut Up and Dance: Youth Culture and Changing Modes of Femininity." *Young* 1 (2): 13–31. https://doi.org/10.1177/110330889300100202.

McWhinney, Tara, and S. Braedley. 2023. "Struggling for Public Services: Lessons from the Saskatchewan Long-term Care Privatization Playbook." *Studies in Political Economy* 104 (2): 93–112. https://doi.org/10.1080/07078552.2023.2234755.

Montei, Amanda. 2023. *Touched Out: Motherhood, Misogyny, Consent, and Control*. Boston: Beacon Press.

Mora, Claudia. 2006. "The Meaning of Womanhood in the Neoliberal Age: Class and Age-Based Narratives of Chilean Women." *Gender Issues* 23: 44–61. https://doi.org/10.1007/s12147-000-0022-1.

Notley, Alice. 1998a. *Mysteries of Small Houses: Poems*. New York: Penguin.

– 1998b. "The Poetics of Disobedience." Paper presented at Contemporary American and English Poetics Conference, Centre of American Studies, King's College, London, 28 February. https://writing.upenn.edu/epc/authors/notley/disob.html.

Oliver, Mary. 1992. *New and Selected Poems*. Boston: Beacon Press.

Onuki, Hironori. 2011. "The Global Migration of Care Labour: Filipino Workers in Japan." In *Feminist Ethics and Social Policy: Towards a New Global Political Economy of Care*, edited by Rianne Mahon and Fiona Robinson, 60–74. Vancouver: UBC Press.

Ostriker, Alicia. 1986. *Stealing the Language: The Emergence of Women's Poetry in America*. Boston: Beacon Press.

Overgaard, Charlotte. 2019. "Rethinking Volunteering as a Form of Unpaid Work." *Nonprofit and Voluntary Sector Quarterly* 48 (1): 128–45. https://doi.org/10.1177/0899764018809419.

Owusu, Prince. 2019. "Racialized Bodies in White Spaces: Exploring Racialization in Long-Term Care Facilities." Paper presented at Take Back Aging: Power, Critique, Imagination Conference, Trent Centre for Aging and Society, Trent University, Peterborough, ON, 28–31 May.

– 2023. "Racialized Workers in White Spaces: Exploring the Experiences of Racialized, Immigrant Care Workers in Rural and Small Town Canadian Long-Term Care Homes." PhD diss., Carleton University. https://doi.org/10.22215/etd/2023-15646.

Palmer, Elyane, and Joan Eveline. 2012. "Sustaining Low Pay in Aged Care Work." *Gender, Work & Organization* 19 (3): 254–75. https://doi.org/10.1111/j.1468-0432.2010.00512.x.

Panitch, Melanie. 2012. *Disability, Mothers, and Organization: Accidental Activists*. New York: Routledge.

Payne, Janna (Klostermann). 2012. "Nesting." *Geez Magazine* 26 (Summer): 28.
– 2013. "How to Speak for God." *The Nashwaak Review* 30–1.
Peltola, Pia, Melissa A. Milkie, and Stanley Presser. 2004. "The 'Feminist' Mystique: Feminist Identity in Three Generations of Women." *Gender & Society* 18 (1): 122–44. https://doi.org/10.1177/0891243203259921.
Pillow, Wanda S. 2003. "Confession, Catharsis, or Cure? Rethinking the Uses of Reflexivity as Methodological Power in Qualitative Research." *Qualitative Studies in Education* 16 (2), 175–96. https://doi.org/10.1080 /0951839032000060635.
Poletti, Anna. 2011. "Coaxing an Intimate Public: Life Narrative in Digital Storytelling." *Continuum Journal of Media & Cultural Studies* 25 (1): 73–83. http://doi.org/10.1080/10304312.2010.506672.
Pratt, Geraldine. 2000. "Research Performances." *Environment and Planning D: Society and Space* 18 (5): 639–51. https://doi.org/10.1068/d218t.
Prentice, Susan, and Pat Armstrong. 2021. "We Must Eliminate Profit-Making from Child Care and Elder Care." *The Conversation*, 25 May. https:// theconversation.com/we-must-eliminate-profit-making-from-child-care -and-elder-care-159407.
Ringrose, Jessica, and Emma Renold. 2010. "Normative Cruelties and Gender Deviants: The Performative Effects of Bully Discourses for Girls and Boys in School." *British Educational Research Journal* 36 (4): 573–96. https://doi .org/10.1080/01411920903018117.
Ringrose, Jessica, and Valerie Walkerdine. 2008. "Regulating the Abject: The TV Make-Over as Site of Neo-Liberal Reinvention toward Bourgeois Femininity." *Feminist Media Studies* 8 (3): 227–46. https://doi.org/10.1080 /14680770802217279.
Rivers-Moore, Megan. 2010. "But the Kids are Okay: Motherhood, Consumption and Sex Work in Neo-Liberal Latin America." *The British Journal of Sociology* 61 (4): 716–36. https://doi.org/10.1111/j.1468-4446 .2010.01338.x. Medline:21138429
Robinson, Fiona. 2011. *The Ethics of Care: A Feminist Approach to Human Security*. Philadelphia, PA: Temple University Press.
– 2019. "Resisting Hierarchies through Relationality in the Ethics of Care." *International Journal of Care and Caring* 4 (1): 11–23. https://doi.org/10.1332 /239788219X15659215344772.
Roll, Rich, host. 2023. "Episode 758 – Zoe Lister-Jones: Creativity, Self-Discovery, and Reinventing Hollywood." *Rich Roll* (podcast). https://www .richroll.com/podcast/zoe-lister-jones-758/
Ruddick, Sara. 1995. *Maternal Thinking: Toward a Politics of Peace*. Boston: Beacon Press.
Santoro, Doris A. 2018. *Demoralized: Why Teachers Leave the Profession They Love and How They Can Stay*. Cambridge, MA: Harvard Education Press.

– 2019. "The Problem with Stories about Teacher 'Burnout.'" *Phi Delta Kappan*101 (4): 26–33. https://doi.org/10.1177/0031721719892971.

Sawchuk, Dana, Janna Klostermann, Laura M. Funk, Maria Cherba, Lauriane Giguère, and Rachel Dunsmore. 2024. "Turned Towards: The Politics of Responsibility in Canadian News Media Narratives of Family Care." *Journal of Canadian Studies* 58 (2): 309–38. https://muse.jhu.edu/pub/50/article/943477.

Sayer, Andrew. 2005. "Class, Moral Worth and Recognition." *Sociology* 39 (5): 947–63. https://doi.org/10.1177/0038038505058376.

Schaffer, Talia. 2019. "Why Lucy Doesn't Care: Migration and Emotional Labor in *Villette.*" *Novel: A Forum on Fiction* 52 (1): 84–106. https://doi.org/10.1215/00295132-7330128.

Schein, Rebecca. 2008. "Landscape for a Good Citizen: The Peace Corps and the Cultural Logics of American Cosmopolitanism." PhD diss., University of California, Santa Cruz.

– 2014. "Hegemony Not Co-Optation: For a Usable History of Feminism." *Studies in Political Economy* 94 (1): 169–76. https://doi.org/10.1080/19187033.2014.11674959.

Shotwell, Alexis. 2013. "'No Proper Feeling for Her House': The Relational Formation of White Womanliness in Shirley Jackson's Fiction." *Tulsa Studies in Women's Literature* 32 (1): 119–41. https://www.jstor.org/stable/43653367.

Siltanen, Janet, Alette Willis, and Willow Scobie. 2009. "Flows, Eddies, Swamps, and Whirlpools: Inequality and the Experience of Work Change." *Canadian Journal of Sociology*34 (4): 1003–32. https://journals.library.ualberta.ca/cjs/index.php/CJS/article/view/3140/5929.

Silverman, Marjorie, Shari Brotman, Marc Molgat, and Elizabeth Gagnon. 2020. "'I've Always Been the One Who Drops Everything': The Lived Experiences and Life-Course Impacts of Young Adult Women Carers." *International Journal of Care and Caring* 4 (3): 331–48. https://doi.org/10.1332/239788220X15859363711424.

Skeggs, Beverley. 2001. "The Toilet Paper: Femininity, Class and Mis-recognition." *Women's Studies International Forum* 24 (3–4): 295–307. https://doi.org/10.1016/S0277-5395(01)00186-8.

– 2004. *Class, Self, Culture.* London: Routledge.

Skinner, Mark W., Alun E. Joseph, and Rachel V. Herron. 2016. "Voluntarism, Defensive Localism and Spaces of Resistance to Health Care Restructuring." *Geoforum* 72: 67–75. https://doi.org/10.1016/j.geoforum.2016.04.004.

Smith, Sidonie, and Julia Watson, eds. 1996. *Getting a Life: Everyday Uses of Autobiography.* Minneapolis: University of Minnesota Press

Somers, Margaret R. 1994. "The Narrative Construction of Identity: A Relational and Network Approach." *Theory and Society* 23 (5): 605–49. https://doi.org/10.1007/BF00992905.

– 2008. *Genealogies of Citizenship: Markets, Statelessness, and the Right to Have Rights*. New York: Cambridge University Press

Stacey, Clare L. 2005. "Finding Dignity in Dirty Work: The Constraints and Rewards of Low-Wage Home Care Labour." *Sociology of Health & Illness* 27 (6): 831–54. https://doi.org/10.1111/j.1467-9566.2005.00476.x. Medline:16283901

– 2011. *The Caring Self: The Work Experiences of Home Care Aides*. Ithaca, NY: Cornell University Press.

Steedman, Carolyn Kay. 1987. *Landscape for a Good Woman: A Story of Two Lives*. New Brunswick, NJ: Rutgers University Press.

Storm, Palle, Susan Braedley, and Sally Chivers. 2017. "Gender Regimes in Ontario Nursing Homes: Organization, Daily Work, and Bodies." *Canadian Journal on Aging* 36 (2): 196–208. https://doi.org/10.1017/s0714980817000071. Medline:28322176

Storm, Palle, and Ruth Lowndes. 2021. "'I Don't Care if They Call Me Black': The Impact of Organisation and Racism in Canadian and Swedish Nursing Homes." *International Journal of Care and Caring* 5 (4): 631–50. http://doi.org/10.1332/239788221X16274947510507.

Streeter, Christine. 2023. "Family Workers: The Work and Working Conditions of Families in Nursing Homes." In *Unpaid Work in Nursing Homes: Flexible Boundaries*, edited by Pat Armstrong, 73–85. Bristol, UK: Policy Press.

– 2024. "The Emotional Economy of Care: Precarious Funding and Structural Violence in Canadian Non-Profit Social Services." PhD diss., Carleton University. https://doi.org/10.22215/etd/2024-16167.

Sutherland, Daniel E. 1981. *Americans and Their Servants: Domestic Service in the United States from 1800 to 1920*. Baton Rouge: Louisiana State University Press.

Syed, Iffath U. 2020. "Racism, Racialization, and Health Equity in Canadian Residential Long Term Care: A Case Study in Toronto." *Social Science & Medicine* 265: 113524. https://doi.org/10.1016/j.socscimed.2020.113524. Medline:33228980

Tamas, Sophia. 2011. *Life After Leaving: The Remains of Spousal Abuse*. New York: Routledge.

Tavory, Iddo. 2016. *Summoned: Identification and Religious Life in a Jewish Neighborhood*. Chicago: University of Chicago Press

Taylor, Judith. (2008). "The Problem of Women's Sociality in Contemporary North American Feminist Memoir." *Gender & Society* 22 (6): 705–27. https://doi.org/10.1177/0891243208324598.

Thomas, Carieta O. 2023. "Technologies of Surveillance: An Intersectional Analysis of Undocumented Caribbean Women Care Workers in the Labour Markets in Canada and the U.S." PhD diss., University of Calgary. https://hdl.handle.net/1880/116865.

Thörn, Håkan, and Sebastian Svenberg. 2016. "'We Feel the Responsibility that You Shirk': Movement Institutionalization, the Politics of Responsibility and the Case of the Swedish Environmental Movement." *Social Movement Studies* 15 (6): 593–609. https://doi.org/10.1080/14742837.2016.1213162.

Toews, Miriam. 2019. *Women Talking*. Toronto: Vintage Canada.

Tronto, Joan C. 1993. *Moral Boundaries: A Political Argument for an Ethic of Care*. New York: Routledge.

– 2013. *Caring Democracy: Markets, Equality, and Justice*. New York: NYU Press.

– 2020. "An Interview with Joan Tronto on Care Ethics and Nursing Ethics." In *Nursing Ethics: Feminist Perspectives*, edited by Helen Kohlen and Joan McCarthy, 93–6. Cham, Switzerland: Springer.

Vanier, Jean. 2002. *From Brokenness to Community*. Mahwa, NJ: Paulist Press.

– 2003. *Finding Peace*. Toronto: House of Anansi Press.

Van Pevenage, Isabelle, Zelda Freitas, Patrik Marier, and Pam Orzeck. 2020. "Are Families Abandoning their Relatives?" In *Getting Wise About Getting Old: Debunking Myths about Aging*, edited by Véronique Billette, Patrik Marier, and Anne-Marie Séguin, 217–24. Vancouver: UBC Press.

Vishmidt, Marina. 2013. "Permanent Reproductive Crisis: An Interview with Silvia Federici." *Mute*, 7 March. https://www.metamute.org/editorial/articles/permanent-reproductive-crisis-interview-silvia-federici.

Visweswaran, Kamala. 1994. *Fictions of Feminist Ethnography*. Minneapolis: University of Minnesota Press.

Vosko, Leah F. 2006. "Precarious Employment: Towards an Improved Understanding of Labour Market Insecurity." In *Precarious Employment: Understanding Labour Market Insecurity in Canada*, edited by Leah Vosko, 3–40. Montreal: McGill-Queen's University Press.

Wajcman, Judy. 2000. "Feminism Facing Industrial Relations in Britain." *British Journal of Industrial Relations* 38 (2): 183–201. https://doi.org/10.1111/1467-8543.00158.

Walker, Margaret Urban. 1997. "Picking Up Pieces: Lives, Stories, and Integrity." In *Feminists Rethink the Self*, edited by Diana T. Meyers, 62–84. New York: Routledge.

Watkins-Hayes, Celeste. 2019. *Remaking a Life: How Women Living With HIV/AIDS Confront Inequality*. Berkeley: University of California Press.

Wells, Paul. 2020. "The Endless Crisis in Ontario's Long-Term Care." *Maclean's*, 27 May. https://www.macleans.ca/politics/the-endless-crisis-in-ontarios-long-term-care/.

Williams, Fiona. 2010. "Claiming and Framing in the Making of Care Policies: The Recognition and Redistribution of Care." UNRISD Gender and Development Programme Paper no. 13. Geneva: UN Research Institute for Social Development. https://digitallibrary.un.org/record/696040.

Winfield, Taylor Paige. 2022a. "All-Encompassing Ethnographies: Strategies for Feminist and Equity-Oriented Institutional Research." *Ethnography* 25 (2): 249–69. https://doi.org/10.1177/14661381221076267.

– 2022b. "Vulnerable Research: Competencies for Trauma and Justice-Informed Ethnography." *Journal of Contemporary Ethnography* 51 (2): 135–70. https://doi.org/10.1177/08912416211017254.

– 2022c. "Interpellative Styles: Choreographies of Identity Disruptions and Repairs." *Sociological Theory* 40 (4): 342–65. https://doi.org/10.1177/07352751221117509.

Winterson, Jeanette. 1996. *Art Objects: Essays on Ecstasy and Effrontery.* Toronto: Vintage Canada.

– 2011. *Why Be Happy When You Could Be Normal?* Toronto: Alfred A. Knopf Canada.

Wood, Helen. 2018. "The Magaluf Girl: A Public Sex Scandal and the Digital Class Relations of Social Contagion." *Feminist Media Studies* 18 (4): 626–42. https://doi.org/10.1080/14680777.2018.1447352.

Wright, Melissa W. 2001. "A Manifesto against Femicide." *Antipode* 33 (3): 550–66. https://doi.org/10.1111/1467-8330.00198. Medline:19165968

Yelin, Hannah. 2016. "'White Trash' Celebrity: Shame and Display." In *Women's Magazines in Print and New Media,* edited by Noliwe Rooks, Victoria Rose Pass, and Ayana K. Weekley, 176–91. New York: Routledge.

Zigon, Jarrett. 2013. "On Love: Remaking Moral Subjectivity in Post-Rehabilitation Russia." *American Ethnologist* 40 (1): 201–15. https://www.jstor.org/stable/23357965.

Zucker, Rachel. 2023. *The Poetics of Wrongness.* Seattle: Wave Books.

Index